SCIENTIFIC AMERICAN *Book*

LIFE and DEATH and MEDICINE

W. H. FREEMAN AND COMPANY
San Francisco

Library of Congress Cataloging in Publication Data

Main entry under title:

Life and death and medicine.

"A Scientific American book."
"Originally appeared as articles in the September
1973 issue of Scientific American."
Includes bibliographies.
1. Medical care—United States. [DNLM: 1. Delivery
of health care—U.S.—Collected works. 2. Medicine—
U.S.—Collected works. WB50 AA1 L7 1973]
RA410.7.L53 616 73-16097
ISBN 0-7167-0892-2
ISBN 0-7167-0891-4 (pbk.)

The thirteen chapters in this book originally appeared
as articles in the September 1973 issue of *Scientific
American.*

Printed in the United States of America

9 8 7 6 5 4 3 2

Paperback edition cover courtesy of the Bettmann
Archive, Inc.

Clothbound edition cover courtesy of New York
Academy of Medicine.

Contents

Foreword

Health is a quality of life enjoyed by entire populations in the rich countries of the world. While this blessing is owed to physical well-being fostered by industrial technology in general, these fortunate peoples look to medicine in particular to supply it. They have been spending on "health care" a rising percentage of their incomes. Drawing upon the on-going revolutionary advances in the life sciences, medicine has returned correspondingly more positive results. The concurrent increase in expenditures and expectations, mutually sustained, has now made medicine, as Kerr L. White observes in the first chapter of this book, "a focus of debate in almost every industrialized society."

In the United States of America the "crisis" in the health services is chronic. It signifies long-term, deep-running changes in the medical economy that are proceeding in the main without direction from plan or policy. The hospital is displacing the physician in the delivery of medical care; the population is displacing the patient as the object of concern; the political process is displacing the market in the allocation of resources. In pragmatic American style, voluntary initiative is joined with public authority to organize the technology of medicine for more effective service.

This book draws the important distinction, often overlooked, between health and medicine. The triptych of chapters following Kerr White's statement of the issues place the finite capacity and role of medicine in the perspective of human biology. Medicine, it turns out, can do little to promote growing up or to prevent growing old and dying. Yet it can secure the natural history of the individual from noxious and hurtful external agents and effects. In the next four chapters the ills that flesh is heir to and the competence of medicine to cope with them are comprehensively surveyed. It is impressive to realize how recent are the advances that have extended to so many people the full experience of human natural history.

How to bring the newly won power of medicine equitably within the reach of all members of· society is the question that occasions this book. The last five chapters consider the social apparatus of American medicine in the stress of accelerating evolution.

The chapters of this book first appeared in the September 1973 issue of SCIENTIFIC AMERICAN, the twenty-fourth in the series of single-topic issues published annually by the magazine. To our colleagues at W. H. Freeman and Company, the book-publishing affiliate of SCIENTIFIC AMERICAN, we declare herewith our appreciation for the enterprise that has made this issue so speedily available in book form.

THE EDITORS*

September 1973

*BOARD OF EDITORS: Gerard Piel (Publisher), Dennis Flanagan (Editor), Francis Bello (Associate Editor), Philip Morrison (Book Editor), Trudy E. Bell, Brian P. Hayes, Jonathan B. Piel, David Popoff, John Purcell, James T. Rogers, Armand Schwab, Jr., C. L. Stong, Joseph Wisnovsky

I

Life and Death and Medicine

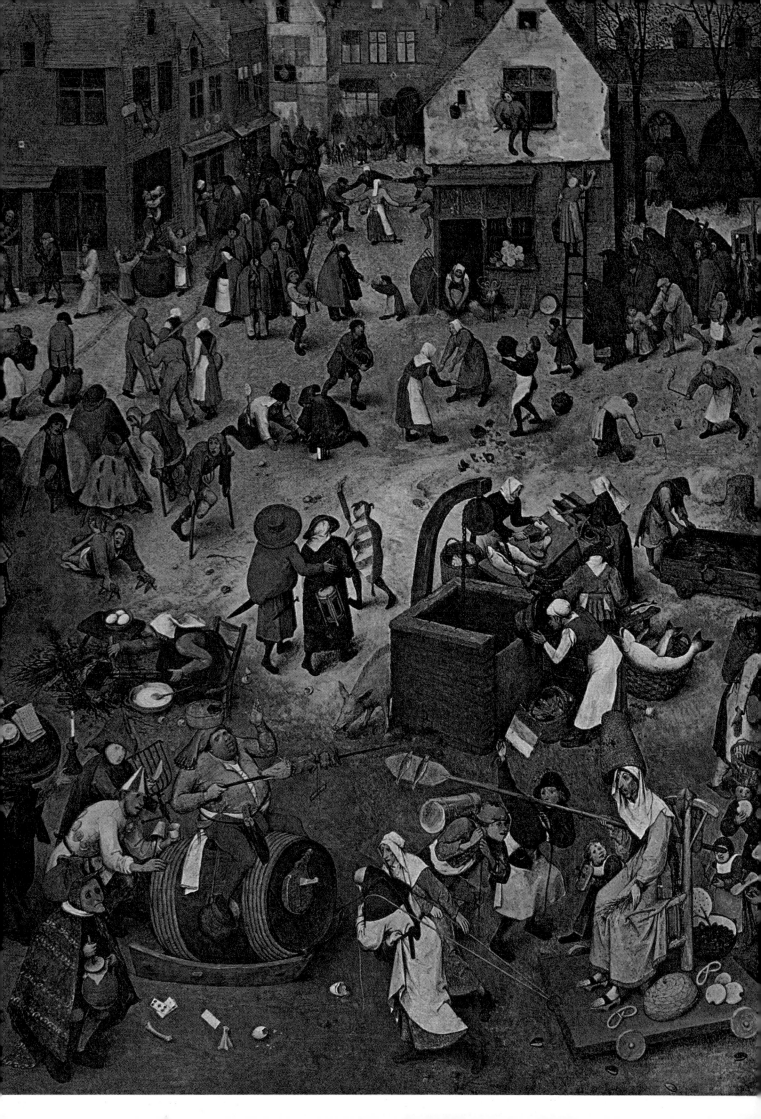

Life and Death and Medicine

KERR L. WHITE

Medicine's success in the treatment of acute illness and injury now makes it possible for it to turn to the promotion of health

Why, at this time, are medicine and the provision of health care rapidly becoming a major focus of debate in almost every industrialized society?

The most obvious reason has to do with the dramatic rise in recent years in the cost of supporting a health-care establishment. The governments and people of the developed countries are understandably becoming concerned about the prospect of spending 8 percent or more of their gross national product on health services. Investments of this magnitude inevitably give rise to questions concerning the relation of value to money: the universal formula for balancing the exchange of energy and resources for benefits.

Part of the reason, however, is to be found in a larger context. A decade of international strife and cultural conflict has challenged the entire spectrum of individual and collective values and has forced the reappraisal of many goals, particularly as they relate to the impact of science and technology on human welfare. The issues of personal accountability and social responsibility, the problems of governance not only of society as a whole but also of its institutions, and the increasingly evident need to establish priorities for allocating energy and resources in all sectors of the economy now dominate discussions of public policy. Medicine is only one arena in which these issues are being debated with growing insight and involvement by concerned consumers, politicians, professionals and scholars.

Two decades of social experimentation promise a more rational basis, derived from the social sciences, for deploying, financing and managing health-care systems more efficiently. So far, however, we have not been outstandingly successful in applying this new knowledge and experience to the problems of organizing health care in the U.S. Inequities and inadequacies in the provision of health care are increasingly apparent, and the burden of health-care expenditures continues to grow.

Three decades of intensive biomedical research have provided a more rational basis for certain elements of medical practice, and as a result there are now many forms of clinical intervention that are clearly more beneficial than they are either harmful or useless. Nonetheless, although disease patterns have changed significantly in the U.S., in part as a result of biomedical advances, there has been little or no improvement in life expectancy for adults since the 1920's. In particular, effective means have not been found for coping with the stubborn complex of chronic and social illnesses that now predominate in the economically advanced countries.

Under these circumstances it is inevitable that society in a period of instability and change should raise basic questions about the contribution of medicine to the quality of personal existence as it is experienced between birth and death. And it is for this reason that the editors of *Scientific American* are presenting a series of articles that discuss medicine in the broadest possible terms: patterns of life, disease and death in human populations; the life history of the individual; the present role of the various kinds of medical intervention and the social, economic and organizational aspects of medical care. In this introduction and in the articles that follow, my colleagues and I shall try to clarify the issues that must be identified, debated and resolved if modern medicine is to make its most beneficial impact on the human condi-

"FIGHT BETWEEN CARNIVAL AND LENT," painted by Pieter Brueghel the Elder in 1559, portrays an allegorical duel between the pre-Lenten spirit of exuberant self-indulgence, symbolized by the stout figure riding on the barrel at lower left, and the Lenten spirit of ascetic self-denial, symbolized by the gaunt figure seated on the wagon at lower right. Brueghel, who excelled at depicting scenes of ordinary life, has included in this painting what can be interpreted as a representation of the full range of human conditions and human activities as they appeared in a 16th-century Flemish town. The painting, only about half of which is reproduced here, is in the Kunsthistorisches Museum in Vienna.

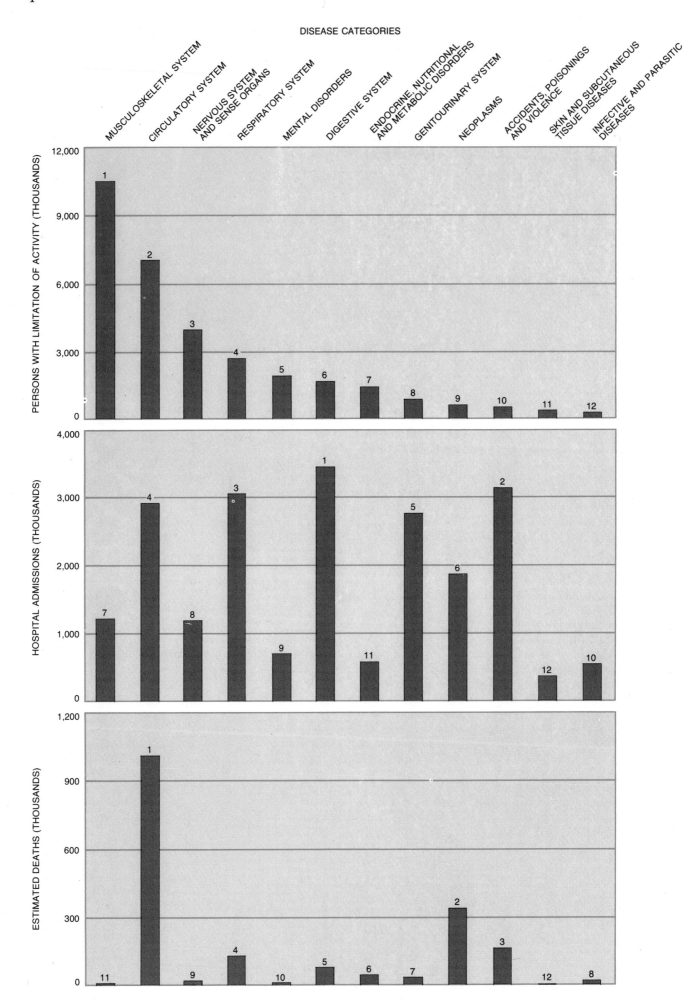

DISEASE CATEGORIES

tion. The issues themselves are not new; only the urgency with which we now perceive them in the U.S. is new.

On what basis does a society assign priorities for medicine? Whose values are expressed in the allocation of a nation's energy and resources to improve the quality of life for all its citizens? At the heart of any consideration for medicine's place in contemporary society are the underlying models that give rise to both assumptions and expectations—assumptions on the part of the health-care establishment about the role of science and technology in the provision of health services, and expectations on the part of consumers about what medicine can accomplish and what they must achieve for themselves by modifying their personal behavior.

Should diseases be likened to ivy growing on the oak tree or are they part of the oak tree itself? Should diseases be regarded as human analogues of defects in an internal-combustion engine or a Swiss watch, or should they be regarded as psychobiological expressions of man evolving within the constraints and potentials contributed from his aliquot of society's gene pool. Are diseases "things" that "happen" to people, or are they manifestations of constructive or destructive relations of individuals in their social and physical environment? Depending on our views about the relevance of these contrasting models for understanding health and disease, we modify our behavior, change our expectations, deploy our resources and measure our accomplishments. By resolving these conflicting views we strike a balance in undergraduate medical education between the biological and the social sciences, in graduate medical education between the preparation of technologically based specialists and psychobiologically trained generalists, in medical organization between solo entrepreneurial practice and multispecialist corporate or group practice, and in medical insurance between "catastrophic" coverage of major medical illnesses and "first dollar" coverage of early am-

bulatory care, anticipatory medicine and counseling.

In the absolute sense there are no right or wrong resolutions of these issues. It is rather the counterbalance of our individual positions as citizens that must determine the social policies affecting the kinds and numbers of health professional we prepare, the facilities and organizations we create and the way we use and finance health care. Above all, our collective position on these issues must determine the contribution of medicine to the quality and duration of our lives and perhaps of our society.

Unwritten social contracts between society and its health-care establishment provide the mandate for physicians and others to minister to individual and collective health needs. In return for the benefits medicine bestows, society accords the health professions substantial power, prestige and pecuniary rewards. Traditionally the overt expression of these contracts has embodied unrealistic promises and expectations. Both parties become increasingly realistic in their renegotiations as they are provided with information about the health needs of people, about the clinical efficacy of preventive and therapeutic procedures, and about the effectiveness and efficiency of different organizational arrangements for providing health care.

Progress in the "old" basic sciences of medicine—anatomy, biochemistry, pathology, pharmacology and physiology— makes it increasingly difficult today for clinical practitioners to invoke tradition and authoritarian pronouncements in support of medical decisions. Progress in the "new" basic sciences of medicine— biostatistics, epidemiology, medical economics and medical sociology—makes it increasingly possible to identify and measure the health problems of individuals and populations and to evaluate the impact of health services on those problems. Both biomedical and health-services research create new insights that reshape our social policies for medical education and medical practice and in turn give rise to another set of issues for research, debate and resolution.

Given the present state of medical science and technology in the context of contemporary industrial communities, what should be the objectives of medical education and medical care? Should medicine adopt the posture that it "fixes" illnesses and "cures" diseases, or should it adopt the posture that it helps people to identify their individual and collective health problems and assists them to resolve or contain them? Should the health-care establishment be judged more on its capacity to investigate and treat abnormal pathology than on its accomplishments in helping patients and their families to understand and manage their problems? What social or even medical utility is to be accorded diagnostic ability if it is not accompanied by effective action and an acceptable outcome? Because we have mastered some procedure, does it follow that society should make it available to all who seek it? To all who can pay for it? To all who need it? Is the new procedure to be preferred over some other form of intervention for the same health problem?

For example, should we concentrate on perfecting coronary-artery bypass operations or on improving early detection and better medical management for patients with coronary-artery insufficiency? Should we concentrate on dialysis and transplants for chronic kidney disease or on early detection, coordinated medical management and follow-up of initial urinary-tract infections? In short, should we continue to develop and rely heavily on complex medical technology for the treatment of acute or life-threatening diseases and conditions? Or would we be better advised to broaden our approach and devote more of our efforts to identifying, containing or resolving the health problems that have major impact on the quality of our lives?

What proportions of society's health-care resources should be directed to the "curing," in contrast to the "caring," components of medical practice? Should resources currently expended on pills, potions and procedures whose benefits or efficacy have never been objectively evaluated be shifted to the provision of personnel and services to make living with chronic disability more comfortable and dying more dignified? How much responsibility has medicine for the terminally ill? What are the limits of these responsibilities, and who decides? Are the decisions determined by scientific knowledge and available technology, or by ethical, social and humanitarian considerations, or by a mixture of both? To what extent should the doctor, in the

STATISTICAL AMBIGUITY at the root of the problem of trying to establish priorities for the allocation of health-care resources in the U.S. is graphically demonstrated in the bar charts on the opposite page, which rank 12 principal disease categories (as defined by the World Health Organization) according to three different measures of ill health. The three measures, all of which are expressed in terms of the number of people affected per year in the U.S., are limitation of activity (*top*), hospital admissions (*middle*) and estimated deaths (*bottom*). The lack of correlation between the respective rank orders is evident. The data on which the illustration is based are for 1971, the latest year for which usable figures for the 12 WHO categories are available from the U.S. National Center for Health Statistics.

original sense of the word, be a teacher of patients and of populations? Is it enough to tell the patient that he has chronic heart failure and prescribe a suitable regimen, or should he and his family be taught to manage the problem so that he can live a satisfying life within the limits of his own capacity without restricting unduly the rights and independence of his family and his community? To what extent should the doctor be responsible for educating his community so that its members can better cope with current epidemics of accidents, alcoholism, delinquency, drug dependency, deprivation, inadequate "parenting," loneliness, occupational boredom and suicide?

Current systems for acquiring and organizing health statistics provide the only available quantitative basis for resolving these issues about the allocation of health resources, and indirectly they condition our basic views on the task of medicine in society. Health and disease are manifested idiosyncratically for each individual as he traverses the hazardous course of life from birth to death. Collectively these experiences with health and disease, with living and dying, find expression as statistics—"people with the tears wiped off," as the medical statistician A. Bradford Hill used to say.

Although imperfect in validity, classification and timeliness, the real limitations of current statistical approaches are associated as much with their orientation and emphasis as with their quality. The problem is best exemplified by the traditional preoccupation of com-

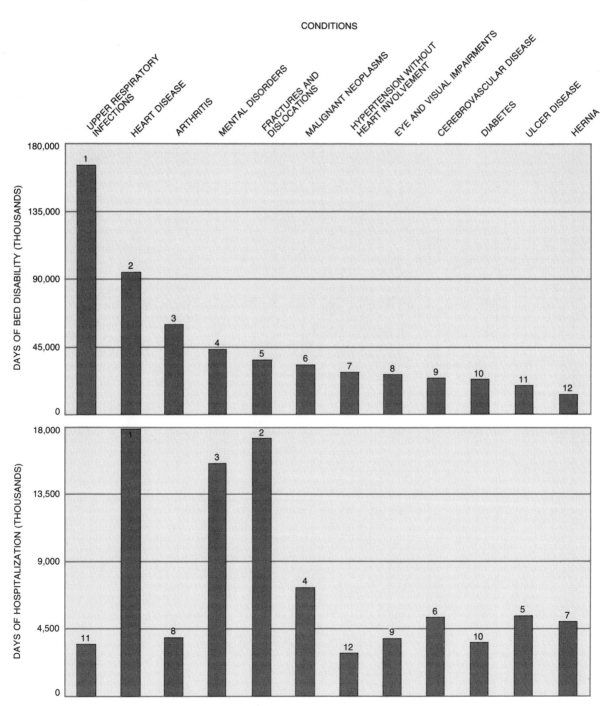

TWO ADDITIONAL MEASURES of the nationwide demand for health services—days of bed disability (*top chart*) and days of hospitalization (*bottom chart*)—focus more specifically on the relative impact of ill health on productivity and the quality of daily life. The 12 principal conditions for which comparative data are available for the U.S. from the National Center for Health Statistics in this case constitute a more refined classification than the 12 WHO disease categories used as the basis of the illustration on page 4.

pilers of vital statistics with death rates (and perhaps in a related way of physicians with dying and postponement of death). Without detracting from the importance of classifying and counting the dead, we should recognize that society is increasingly concerned with the problems of living, the quality of life and the burden of disability, distress and dependency.

For example, even the concept of "disease," based on an anatomical and clinical classification introduced a century and a half ago, may be disappearing. The more we learn about the genetic and molecular substrates of disease and the interacting forces arising from within and without the individual, the harder it becomes to classify ill health into discrete categories. The International Classification of Diseases, developed under the auspices of the World Health Organization and adapted for use in the U.S. by the National Center for Health Statistics, is devoted primarily to classifying and coding causes of death rather than categorizing illness. It has limited utility for hospital care and is largely unsuited for classifying health problems associated with ambulatory care, limitation of activity or bed disability. Patients describe complaints, problems and symptoms, not diseases, when they first perceive themselves to be ill and seek care. "Disease" and its classification are professional constructs, whereas "health problems and complaints" are lay constructs, and we need to recognize the differences in developing our health-information systems.

The problem of relating health-care priorities and resources to the relative impact of disability, disease and death can be illustrated by referring to the latest available data on three parameters of health and disease for 12 of the 17 principal WHO categories for which usable figures are available [*see illustration on page 4*]. The illustration ranks the causes of limitation of activity, as perceived by respondents to a national household-interview survey. "Limitation of activity" is defined as inability or decreased ability to carry on the usual activities for one's age-sex group, such as working, keeping house, going to school and participating in civic, church and recreational activities. It is largely a measure, from the individual's point of view, of the long-term burden of chronic disease and impairment, and indirectly of morbidity in relation to the quality of life. "Hospital admissions" are probably the best currently available measure of disease as recognized and defined by the medical profession; since only a small

proportion of the population have more than one admission a year, these figures essentially represent people with hospital admissions in 1971. The rank orders for these two measures bear little relation to each other. When compared with the rank order for "Deaths," the third and most widely used measure, there is even less correlation; many categories that generate substantial volumes of disability and disease produce comparatively few deaths.

The allocation of health-care resources should be related to two additional measures. "A day of bed disability" is one during which a person stays in bed for more than half of the daylight hours because of a specific acute or chronic illness or injury. "Days of hospital care" are a subset of bed-disability days and reflect the intensity of demand for health services.

Let us now consider the 12 principal conditions for which comparative data are available on days of bed disability and days of hospital care [*see illustration on opposite page*]. These conditions constitute a more refined classification than the 12 principal disease categories in the illustration on page 4 and reflect more specifically the relative impact of ill health on productivity and the quality of daily life. Apart from funds devoted to fundamental laboratory research, which is a priceless prerequisite for most advances in medical science, figures for money spent on clinical research and care for each of these conditions are not available. If they were, however, they should reflect some coherent relation between health resources needed or consumed and disability and disease experienced by the citizens of the U.S. For example, if we accord relief of disability, disease and death about equal priority, we would allocate more money to heart disease than to cancer (malignant neoplasms). If disability alone had a high priority, arthritis and the musculoskeletal category could be near the top.

None of these measures is entirely satisfactory in orientation, quality, definition or classification if our object is to improve the decision-making process for the allocation of resources, and particularly if we give priority to the problems of living in contrast to those of dying. Conspicuously lacking, for example, is reliable information about the number of people seeking ambulatory care for their health problems. Here the contrast between the problems of daily living and the problems of dying is undoubtedly more pronounced.

The most reliable information available on this question is a compilation of

the 12 most common conditions treated by 171 general practitioners in England and Wales in 1958 [*see illustration on next page*]. Problems of classification make it difficult to relate these conditions to the major causes of death, but we can at least say that the common cold is not one of them and very few of the general practitioner's patients will die of the conditions for which they visit him most frequently.

Similar data for the U.S. are not available, but that deficiency is being remedied by the National Center for Health Statistics. A national probability sample of physicians in office-based practice, who will fill out short encounter forms on their patients for a period of one week, will relate problems, complaints and symptoms to diagnoses, tests, treatments, referrals and disposition. The importance of this annual survey for defining the objectives of undergraduate and graduate medical education, of health-manpower training and of supporting facilities, equipment and services can hardly be overemphasized.

Health data for small areas such as counties, standard metropolitan statistical areas and even states are also largely lacking, but this too is being tackled through the development of cooperative statistical systems involving Federal, state and local participation. In both the short run and the long we cannot make sensible decisions about professional education and the cost-benefit ratio of medical services and research without vastly improved health information on the problems of living as well as the probabilities of death [see "The Ills of Man," by John H. Dingle, page 49].

Many of these issues concerning the priorities of medicine are finding contemporary expression in the growth, even renaissance, of primary care and the general practitioner, or family doctor, in North America and Europe. As we have seen, no reliable estimates are available on the distribution in populations of health problems, symptoms and complaints brought to physicians at the initial time of contact, and only limited estimates are available on the medical reasons for using hospitals or long-term-care facilities. In the absence of such elementary "marketing" information it is virtually impossible to define the overall objectives of medical education, to apportion opportunities for training physicians of all types in accordance with need, or to determine the best balance of health-care facilities and services. There is a growing consensus, however, that in the U.S. primary care has been largely neglected in favor of specialty care, that in the United Kingdom the quality of primary care needs substantial improvement, and that in many other European countries the coordination of primary care with other levels of care in some viable form of regionalization is essential to achieve optimal use of all resources. This is particularly true of expensive, technologically based resources provided by hospitals and other health-care facilities that need to be used prudently, promptly and appropriately.

In many ways the need for primary medical care can be considered the central problem facing American medicine today. Two schools of thought illustrate the issues. The first sees the physician's task as being concerned essentially, if not solely, with diseases for which there are recognized treatments or palliative measures (or diseases that, if they were investigated more intensively, might eventually be better understood and treated). The trivial, commonplace, chronic and terminal problems should be

identified and managed by other health personnel. These "physician-extenders" (physician assistant, nurse practitioner and health associate are among the titles currently used) should have largely technical training, be supported by technological devices and be guided by prescribed instructions telling them how to make decisions. They should receive various degrees of supervision and surveillance by a physician. This physician's own training in primary medical care is as a rule only vaguely specified, and po-

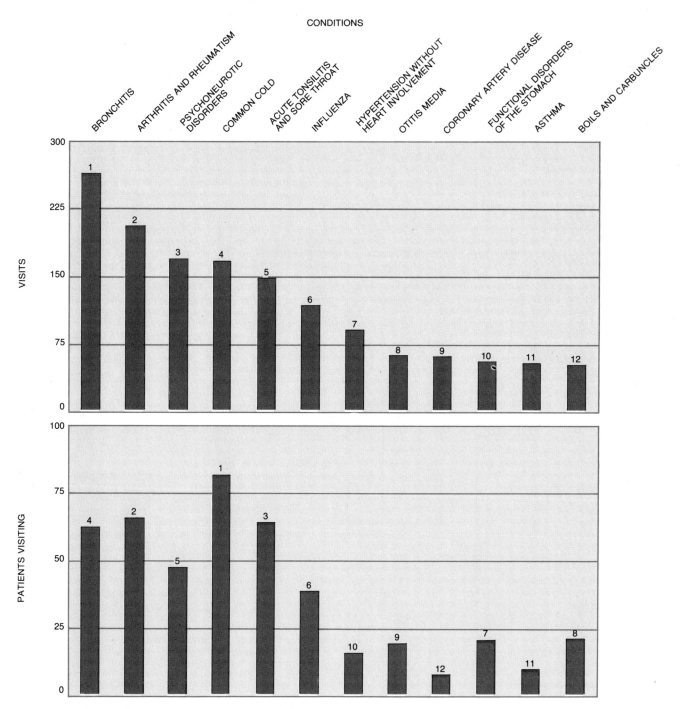

THE MOST RELIABLE INFORMATION available about the number of people seeking ambulatory care for their health problems is represented by this compilation of the 12 most common conditions (per 1,000 people) treated by 171 general practitioners in England and Wales in 1958. Such health data, which give priority to the problems of living in contrast to those of dying, are not available for the U.S. but are clearly needed if the decision-making process for the allocation of health-care resources is to be improved.

tential students are usually described as not finding the problems of primary care very interesting. (Presumably patients find them more so.) Patients should be referred to the supervising physician or to a specialist if the primary-care physician-extender is unsuccessful (according to his own lights) in identifying or managing the patient's problems. This scheme for the provision of primary care was conceived and is being advocated by the leadership of the American academic medical community and by hospital-based, technologically oriented specialists. Few advocates of these arrangements have themselves had any direct, extensive experience with the provision of continuing primary care to general populations.

The second school sees the task of medicine as being concerned with helping patients and families to identify and manage their own health problems, indeed to work toward the full achievement of their own potential for personal growth. Health problems in this context are regarded as essentially problems of living constructively and dying more comfortably without imposing intolerable burdens on oneself and others. They constitute the vast bulk of medical problems presented by patients to sources of primary care and are regarded as responses to the stresses and strains of domestic, occupational and social life and such potentially noxious contemporary accompaniments of industrialized societies as foul air, noise, cigarette smoking, chemical contaminants, constant residential mobility, jet-travel fatigue, radiation hazards, urban crowding and traffic congestion.

Most of these problems have a behavioral component and tend to be observed first by the pediatrician, for whom they constitute the majority of contemporary complaints. They are viewed as requiring a broadly educated physician, selected initially for his interest in people, his "caring" qualities, his capacity for integrating a vast array of usable knowledge from the biomedical and social sciences, his interest in resolving problems as well as in analyzing their genesis, his ability to tolerate anxiety and to make decisions in the face of uncertainty and his capacity for working with the open-ended nature of the problems of living and dying that most patients present most of the time.

This primary-care physician should be well trained scientifically, particularly in the behavioral sciences. He should know the limits of his capabilities and have access to teams of highly trained subspecialists supported by ancillary personnel, by technologically sophisticated equipment and particularly by on-line computer regimes that provide timely information about the distribution of clinical manifestations and the efficacy of treatments. This scheme has its origins in the efforts of the academic and professional societies that have rejuvenated primary medical care under the aegis of family medicine in the U.S. and general practice in the United Kingdom, the Netherlands and Canada. Most advocates of this definition of medicine's task have had experience in the practice of primary care, and some have done extensive research in the field. Until recently few such people have been regarded as acceptable candidates for medical-school faculties in any country.

These two schools represent polar views of medicine's task and illustrate the basic issues at stake in the current process of redefining medicine's mandate. The first is unlikely to be successful because it confuses the nature of the medical-care process and the characteristics of the information needed for most clinical decision making. At the level of primary care decisions about the severity, complexity and urgency of the patient's illness are based on a probabilistic system, not a deterministic one. The decision maker needs to be skilled in eliciting information from the patient and in interpreting vast amounts of data on the prevalence and patterns of clinical manifestations in general populations. The best that contemporary medical science can offer requires that these two sets of information be put together intelligently. At this juncture the task of the primary physician requires judgment, wisdom, compassion, patience and common sense, not more hardware. Decision making in medicine is rarely simple even in so-called simple cases. To assume otherwise is to misjudge the task of medicine and the power of organized medical knowledge and medical care. It is rare that specific decisions for individual patients can be found in books or made by computers.

Resolution of these conflicting viewpoints poses a major challenge to the medical profession. In the final analysis the terms of the unwritten contract depend largely on the profession's own capacity for generating new knowledge about health problems and for providing new forms of leadership on behalf of the society it serves.

As the postindustrial society emerges and demands to produce more goods are replaced by demands to provide improved services, medicine is faced with yet another set of problems and related issues. Traditionally the physician has been taught to direct all his skills and attention to the individual patients who consult him. He receives his training in teaching hospitals, where the complaint-response system prevails and the focus is largely on acute, episodic illnesses that are usually serious and that can be cured or effectively palliated. This limited exposure of young physicians and their teachers to the full range of ordinary and complex health problems generated by large general populations, and their intense preoccupation with only those patients who are selected to obtain care in teaching hospitals, leave enormous qualitative and quantitative gaps in their experience and inevitably condition their views about the tasks of contemporary medicine.

The dimensions of the problem can be illustrated by considering the distribution of demand for medical care by a typical population of 1,000 persons in one year [*see illustration on next page*]. As the illustration shows, the vast bulk of care is provided by physicians in ambulatory settings. Only 10 percent of the people are admitted to a hospital and only 1 percent to a university hospital where the young physician is trained. The discrepancies between the world of medical practice and that of medical education are more than those of town and gown. They are discrepancies of experience, responsibility, functions and scale.

A belated recognition in the U.S. of the issues confronting medicine with respect to both the overall content of medical practice and the related objectives of professional education is now broadening to a concern for the ways in which medical care is best organized to meet society's needs. Although the individual patient-physician relationship remains the central element in medical care, the profession is gradually acknowledging a larger collective responsibility for the health of the entire community—not the sole responsibility, but a major responsibility. If society has health problems, to whom should it turn if not to its health-care establishment? In former times an artificial dichotomy, professionally conceived, institutionalized and perpetuated, existed between "private medicine" and "public health." No longer does it appear sensible to separate preventive care from curative and restorative care, or the public's health from the individual's health. These are attitudinal, professional and institutional anachronisms for which there is no basis in contemporary knowledge or need.

How should the profession organize its efforts so that it can promote optimal health for all individuals within the limits of the resources society is willing to provide? Again we could come to grips more successfully with the basic issues of priorities and value for money if we had adequate information about the distribution of problems in populations and communities. But experience and logic can at least suggest guides for sensible choices.

There are, broadly speaking, three categories of health problems. First there are those with a very low probability of being experienced by any one individual in his lifetime but with a relatively definable and predictable prevalence for large general populations of from 500,-000 to several million. Examples include certain congenital abnormalities, unusual genetic and molecular aberrations, certain malignant neoplasms, catastrophic trauma, rare metabolic and endocrine disorders, acute poisonings,

complex immune reactions and diseases acquired by travelers in areas remote from home. These problems require what is usually described as tertiary care: highly specialized, technologically based intensive care centralized in large medical centers and frequently located in universities.

Second, there are problems for which the probability is still low for a given individual but the prevalence is more substantial in general populations. It usually takes a population of from 25,000 to several hundred thousand to generate definable demands for health services. These problems include industrial, agricultural and traffic accidents, burns, fractures, tumors requiring radiation therapy, selected cardiac disorders, and emergencies needing uncommon types of blood or unusual laboratory tests. They require what is called secondary care: specialized consultant care that should be based in large-sized community hospitals (or district hospitals, to use the European term).

The third category of health problems

includes those with a high probability of affecting any one individual at least once, if not frequently, in the course of a lifetime. They include respiratory infections, common forms of heart disease, arthritis, asthma, obesity, visual impairments, gastrointestinal disturbances, minor accidents and emotional problems. Comparatively small populations, ranging from 1,000 to 25,000, produce enough of these everyday problems to keep a general physician and his supporting personnel fully occupied. It is these problems, when they are not managed through self-care by the family, that require primary care: treatment based in offices, clinics, ambulatory facilities or health centers with a few "holding," or observation, beds close to where people live and work.

These three fundamentally different patterns of disease in general populations have important implications for the organization of health services, particularly in combination with the fact that most patients seek care initially not for specific diseases but for nonspecific health problems, complaints or symptoms. For the problems that require tertiary care both the low prevalence rates and the highly specialized and expensive resources required for effective management dictate the centralization of services. Only a fairly large community can afford the resources required and at the same time ensure reasonable equity of access for all its members to services of uniformly high quality. For many communities and regions the services are so specialized and expensive that only one source for such care is feasible; larger populations may be able to afford several sources, but even here unlimited choice is increasingly regarded as being wasteful. The same arguments apply to the secondary-care problems, but since they are more prevalent and the resources less costly, more choices are possible and greater dispersion is desirable.

For the class of primary-care health problems, however, multiple sources of care are possible and indeed essential if choice and constructive competition are values we want to preserve and encourage. For these common problems prompt and equitable access to a full range of health-care services is a matter of high priority in industrialized societies. This can be most readily achieved by numerous and widely dispersed health centers, clinics and physicians' offices, clustered around community or district hospitals and supported by links to sources of up-to-date information, consultation and highly specialized care.

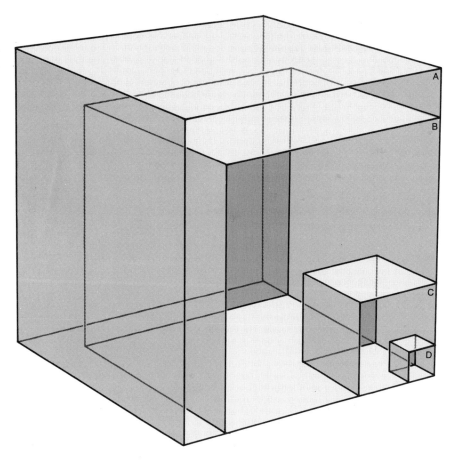

DISTRIBUTION OF DEMAND for medical care by a typical population in one year (1970), represented volumetrically in this illustration, points up the discrepancy in scale between the world of medical practice and the world of medical education in the U.S. Out of a total population at risk of 1,000 (*cube A*), an average of 720 people visited a physician in an ambulatory setting at least once (*cube B*), 100 people were admitted to a hospital at least once (*cube C*) and only 10 were admitted to a university hospital at least once (*cube D*).

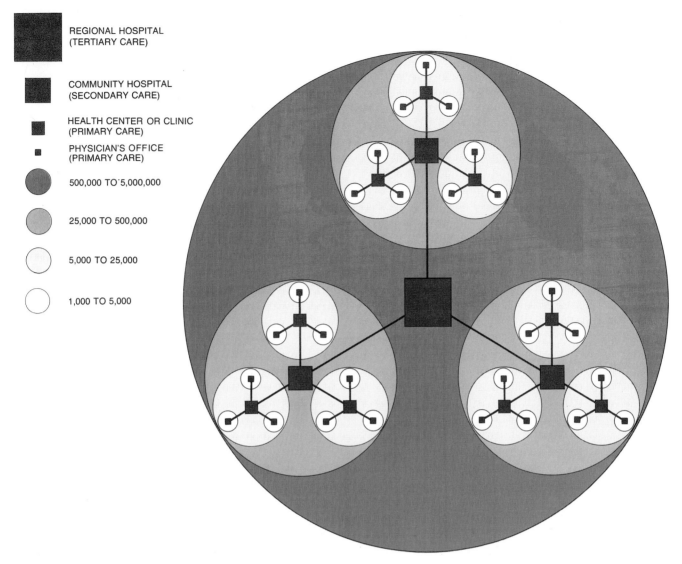

REGIONAL HOSPITAL
(TERTIARY CARE)

COMMUNITY HOSPITAL
(SECONDARY CARE)

HEALTH CENTER OR CLINIC
(PRIMARY CARE)

PHYSICIAN'S OFFICE
(PRIMARY CARE)

500,000 TO 5,000,000

25,000 TO 500,000

5,000 TO 25,000

1,000 TO 5,000

WELL-DEFINED HIERARCHY exists between the three levels of medical care (primary, secondary and tertiary) in countries where health services are regionalized. The effect of such regionalization is suggested by this illustration, which indicates the type of health-care facility associated with each level of care and the average population served by each facility (*key at left*). Tertiary care is usually defined as highly specialized, technologically based intensive care centralized in large medical centers and frequently located in universities; secondary care is somewhat less specialized consultant care based in fairly large community, or district, hospitals; primary care is treatment based in physicians' offices, clinics, ambulatory facilities or health centers close to where people live and work.

Recourse to the sources of primary care, in other words, should put a patient in reach of secondary and tertiary care promptly and reliably if it turns out to be necessary.

In countries where health services are regionalized there is a well-established hierarchical relation between the three levels of care [*see illustration above*]. In many settings regional relations are based on statutory or centrally administered mandates and associated regulations.

In the U.S. we are faced with the difficult task of organizing our resources so that the economic and medical benefits of regionalization can be realized without sacrificing the equally desirable benefits associated with a reasonable choice of a primary physician. Somewhere be-

tween the extremes of a monolithic national health service and the fragmented arrangements that currently prevail in the U.S., with their consequent uneven quality and accessibility, a balance must be struck.

Similarly, some compromise must be reached between those who believe the only opportunity for the entrepreneur in health care is in solo, even isolated, clinical practice and those who consider a large national system to be the best way to organize and administer health care. New organizational patterns must emerge and there are many possibilities. They range from loose contractual affiliations among solo practitioners and small partnerships of primary physicians, community hospitals and subspecialty medical centers, on the one hand,

and on the other, to large competitive local, regional or national systems—even "bureaucracies"—operating under government, voluntary, public or private auspices.

Among the possible options the one unique contribution of American medicine to the organization of health care deserves particular attention: prepaid comprehensive group practice. This arrangement constitutes the prototype for the health-maintenance organization (HMO) now espoused in many quarters. The essential elements of this organizational arrangement include prepayment of fixed annual premiums or taxes for each person or family enrolled, a contractual relation between the enrollees and the health-care plan or the providers for an agreed set of benefits, and an or-

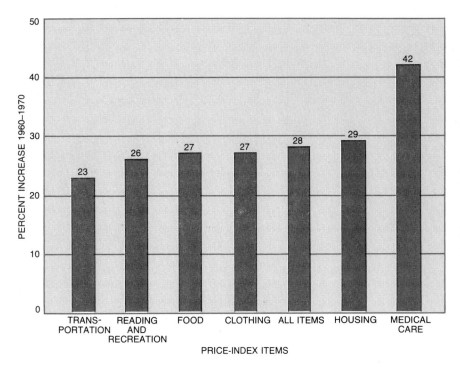

DRAMATIC RISE in recent years in the cost of supporting a health-care establishment in an industrialized society is put into perspective in this chart, which compares the percent increase in the cost of medical care in the U.S. with other major components in the consumer price index for the decade 1960–1970. The chart is adapted from one in a recently published book, *Dynamics of Health and Disease*, by Carter L. Marshall and David Pearson.

ganized multispecialty group of physicians and other health professionals compensated by annual salaries and related incentives. The entire organization is at professional and financial risk for the provision of a full range of health-care services, including ambulatory and hospital care at all three levels.

The trick in the U.S. will be to encourage the evolution of health-care arrangements and organizations that give reasonable choices to both consumers and physicians, that provide responsive and responsible services at reasonable rates and that meet established standards for quality and equity of access. It is difficult to see how we can achieve these new arrangements in the foreseeable future without some Federal leadership and financing. External monitoring of quality and some form of regulation through franchising and in some instances subsidy, depending on the form of national health insurance that eventually emerges, seem inevitable. The professional-standards-review organizations represent only the beginning of Federal, state and local monitoring of the quality of medical care.

In addition attention will have to be paid to the urgent need for adequate capitalization of new health-care organizations and institutions. The entire system is at present labor-intensive and undercapitalized. The possibilities for accomplishing its adequate capitalization include philanthropy, Federal and state grants or loans, debt and equity financing. Whatever its source, the new capital will have to be amortized over a couple of decades and must be paid for by the consumers and taxpayers. Although the notion of "profit" in medicine is confused with the concept of "incentive" and has been regarded as unwholesome if not unethical in some circles, the logical basis for this position is difficult to discern. As in the communications and transportation systems in the U.S., or even in the competitive national and private airline bureaucracies in Canada and the United Kingdom, there may well be a place for profit-making health-care systems. Such systems can mobilize private capital and can effectively take advantage of economies of scale while preserving some of the entrepreneurial spirit of solo practice. Of necessity they must undertake adequate "marketing" studies, assume "risks" and provide consumer satisfaction. Although privately owned, they probably have to be widely held public companies with expert management in order to generate adequate capital. If such systems cannot meet established standards for the quality and the distributional equity of services, or if they go bankrupt, they can always be taken over by nonprofit organizations or by local or state governments. In that event the health problems, the patients and the personnel will remain; only the ownership and the control will change.

At present we simply do not know whether particular forms of ownership, particular types of control or particular styles of management for health-care institutions or systems can be associated with differences in the health-care status of the patients who patronize them. Opportunities abound for comparison, experiment and creative innovation. This remains one of the challenges and opportunities for health care in the U.S. What is clear is that containment of our overall health-care costs within tolerable limits will be difficult without expert management of those systems. At present our hospitals and health-care institutions are largely run by amateurs with on-the-job training. For example, no more than a third of the country's 17,500 hospital administrators have had anything that can be regarded as formal training for managing these complex organizations.

New financial incentives, particularly the notions of prebudgeting based on fixed annual payments for each person enrolled in a health-care plan or system and of assigned risk or responsibility, should encourage needed changes. For example, prepaid group practices (such as the Kaiser Foundation Health Plan and the Health Insurance Plan of Greater New York) have already demonstrated that a large portion of the health-care dollar can be shifted from inpatient hospital care to other modalities of care, particularly to ambulatory care.

Although the eventual patterns of organization in the U.S. and the extent of Federal involvement are still obscure, there will undoubtedly be a growing need for quasipublic authorities on the regional, state or community levels to monitor the type and quality of care their citizens receive, to franchise, license or certify health-care organizations, services and facilities, and to review costs and approve premiums, rates, charges and benefit packages for health-care plans and institutions. That in turn is unlikely to happen without effective financial incentives and a combination of Federal regulation, surveillance and control.

Health-care systems in even the most developed countries are in a rudimentary stage of evolution compared with systems for the mass production of manufactured goods and agricultural products or even for the provision of services such as transportation, communications and defense. In most service systems one can identify examples where optimal mixtures of science, technology, capital, personnel and management are meeting the needs of defined markets or populations effectively and efficiently to the satisfaction of most people most of the time. In the U.S. the same can rarely be said for health care as yet.

One element that is clearly missing is a first-rate medical intelligence service to analyze quantitative information bearing on health-care issues in the light of political, social and economic factors. To accomplish this we need groups of policy analysts at Federal and state levels of government and in extragovernmental institutes and universities. To the extent that history and experiences here and abroad, together with information and critical thought, can illuminate health-care problems and issues, policy analysis should be encouraged, if not required. How else can we take advantage of the opportunities afforded by our traditions of diversity and pluralism, by the advances in science and technology and by the American talent for organization? There is no greater challenge in the realm of social services than the application of these powerful forces to improving our health-care arrangements.

In all our efforts we should not forget that health is a personal matter and an individual responsibility, that we are born alone and we die alone. There is a limit to the extent that collective action can reverse the ravages of time, ameliorate the human condition or forestall our ultimate death. Insofar as knowledge can help, however, we should pursue it vigorously and use it sensibly—knowledge not only about our psychobiological system but also about ourselves and our relations to one another, knowledge about social, political and economic forces that shape our future, and knowledge about the health-care resources, professions and institutions that seek to improve our common lot. It is more science in medicine, not less, that will ultimately help to improve the quality of life and ease the perilous adventure from birth to death.

LEVELS OF MEDICAL CARE are characterized loosely in this illustration according to the relative importance of primary, secondary or tertiary care in dealing with a wide range of medical problems and functions. The more important the level of care, the darker the color in the appropriate box.

FUNCTION	RELATIVE CONTENT		
	PRIMARY CARE	SECONDARY CARE	TERTIARY CARE
HEALTH PROBLEM			
RARE AND COMPLICATED			
INFREQUENT AND SPECIFIC			
COMMON AND NONSPECIFIC			
SITE OF CARE			
AMBULATORY CARE			
INPATIENT: GENERAL CARE			
INPATIENT: INTENSIVE CARE			
REFERRAL PATTERN			
DIRECT ACCESS			
REFERRAL PRACTICE			
EXTENT OF RESPONSIBILITY			
CONTINUING CARE			
INTERMITTENT CARE			
EPISODIC CARE			
INFORMATION SOURCE			
PATIENT AND FAMILY			
EPIDEMIOLOGICAL DATA BASE			
BIOMEDICAL DATA BASE			
USE OF TECHNOLOGY			
COMPLEX EQUIPMENT AND STAFF			
REGULAR LABORATORY AND X-RAY			
OFFICE LABORATORY			
ORIENTATION			
PREVENTION AND HEALTH MAINTENANCE			
EARLY DIAGNOSIS AND DISABILITY CONTAINMENT			
PALLIATION AND REHABILITATION			
TRAINING NEEDED			
BROAD AND GENERAL			
CONCENTRATED			
NARROW AND HIGHLY SPECIALIZED			

II

Growing Up

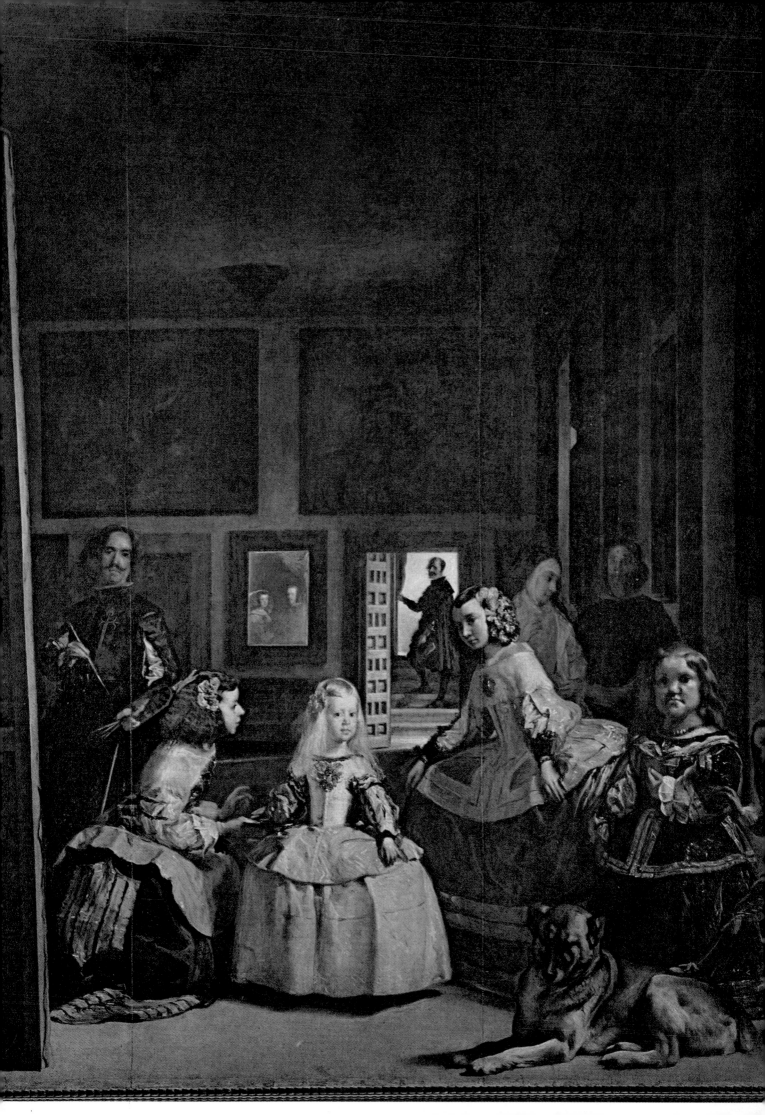

Growing Up

J. M. TANNER

Events in the interaction between the environment and the genetic potential during the growth of the child are critical to the health of the adult. At the same time "normal" growth is highly variable

Over the past 100 years there has been a deep change in attitudes toward the years of childhood, following the realization of how crucial the process of growing up is to the entire subsequent life of the individual. Instead of child labor we have universal education; instead of birch rods we have psychotherapists. The study of child growth and development is central to modern educational theory and practice. It also bears heavily on social policy concerning the distribution of food, the condition of housing and the control of population. The study of growth in this context has made us appreciate more than ever before the intricate way in which genetic endowment and cultural forces continuously interact to mold the life of the individual child. For example, what are we to make of the fact that in most industrial countries the age of menarche (first menstruation) has shown a steady downward trend of three to four months per decade for the past century? Identical twins growing up in the same environment attain menarche within a month or two of each other, so that the

genes are clearly involved. Yet the trend suggests that the environmental factors can exert a powerful influence.

There are two ways of plotting a child's growth. One is to simply show the child's height at successive ages. Another is to show the increments of height gained from one age to the next, expressed as the rate of growth per year. If we think of growth as a form of motion, the first curve shows the distance traveled and the second shows the velocity of growth. The velocity curve reflects the child's state at any particular time better than the distance curve, because the distance curve depends largely on how much the child has grown in the preceding years. Children of the same age show a wide variation in their height. In fact, this variation is so great that if a child who was of exactly average height at his seventh birthday grew not at all for two years, he would still be just within the normal limits of height attained at age nine.

In general the velocity of growth decreases from the fourth month of fetal life until the early teen-age years. At that

time there is a marked acceleration of growth called the adolescent growth spurt. The adolescent spurt is a constant feature in all human growth curves. On the average it comes two years earlier in girls than in boys. It is less pronounced in girls because it is caused partly by testosterone, the male sex hormone.

Human growth itself is a rather regular process. Contrary to opinions still heard occasionally, growth in height does not proceed by fits and starts, nor does growth in upward dimensions alternate with growth in transverse dimensions. The more carefully the measurements are made, the more regular the succession of points in the graph of a child's growth becomes. A good technique of positioning the child for measurement is as important as the proper apparatus for accurately measuring his height. Careful positioning minimizes the decrease in height that occurs during the day for postural reasons. The decrease is significant: it can be as much as three centimeters with a bad positioning technique but is less than half a centimeter with good technique.

Mathematical curves have been fitted with great success to measurements of individuals followed during the adolescent spurt. Not only the height of the children has been fitted in this way but also the length of the arms, legs and trunk and the width of the shoulders and hips. Such serial studies of individuals are called longitudinal, as opposed to the studies of populations called cross-sectional, in which each child is measured only once.

The average boy is slightly taller than the average girl until the girl's adolescent spurt begins. Between the ages of about 11 and 13 the average girl is taller. Moreover, she is also heavier, in most

"LAS MENINAS" ("THE MAIDS OF HONOR"), painted by Diego Velazquez in 1656, shows among other things three conditions of human growth. At left center in the portion of the painting reproduced on the opposite page is the Infanta Margarita Maria, the daughter of Philip IV of Spain and his second wife, Marianna of Austria. The Infanta is a normal child of five. (She is dressed as a miniature adult, which reflects a difference in attitudes toward children between then and now.) The two figures at the far right are dwarfs. The woman suffers from achondroplasia, in which the growth of the trunk is normal but the limbs are stunted and the face is characteristically altered. The man, who appears to be a child with his foot playfully on the back of the dog, suffers from the principal form of dwarfism: isolated growth-hormone deficiency. In this form of dwarfism growth is severely limited but the proportions of the body are normal. The Infanta later married Leopold I, the Holy Roman Emperor. Her mother and father appear in the picture as reflections in the mirror to the left of the man in the illuminated doorway. Velazquez, who painted the scene as though he were making a portrait of the king and queen while the Infanta looked on, put himself in the picture at the far left. The painting has a room to itself at the Prado in Madrid.

respects as strong and sexually much more mature. Only when the boy's spurt begins does he pass the girls, to take up his adult status of being the larger and more physically powerful sex. This changeover in size and maturity in the sexes is just one example of how the biology of growth presents problems in the organization of activities in schools.

Nearly all the bones and muscles take part in the adolescent growth spurt. The increase in the size of the muscles is much more marked in boys than in girls. This growth, perhaps combined with changes in the muscles themselves toward more power per unit of cross-sectional area of muscle, results in a large increase in the strength of adolescent boys. Boys also develop a larger heart and lungs in relation to their size than girls. In addition they develop a higher systolic blood pressure, a lower rate of heartbeat while they are resting, a greater capacity for oxygen in the blood and a greater power for neutralizing the chemical products of muscular exercise (such as lactic acid), resulting in a faster rate of recovery from physical exhaustion.

At the same time the male's shoulders show a proportionally greater spurt in width than the female's, while the female's hips widen more than the male's. In short, at adolescence the male becomes more adapted for the tasks of hunting, fighting and manipulating heavy objects, as is necessary in some forms of food gathering. It is as a direct result of these anatomical and physiological changes that athletic ability increases to such a marked degree in boys at adolescence. The notion of a boy outgrowing his strength at this stage has little observational support. Strength, athletic skill and physical endurance all progress rapidly throughout adolescence; if the adolescent feels weak and becomes easily exhausted, it is for psychological and social reasons.

Important sex differences develop in the individual long before puberty. During prenatal life the Y chromosome of the male induces the growth of the testes. These organs manufacture testosterone, the hormone that causes the development of the external male genitalia. In addition fetal testosterone has a specific action on the hypothalamic portion of the brain, transforming it into a male hypothalamus. The action is irrevocable, at least in experimental animals, and has to happen during a short period when the hypothalamus is particularly sensitive. If no testosterone is received during that period, the hypothalamus differen-

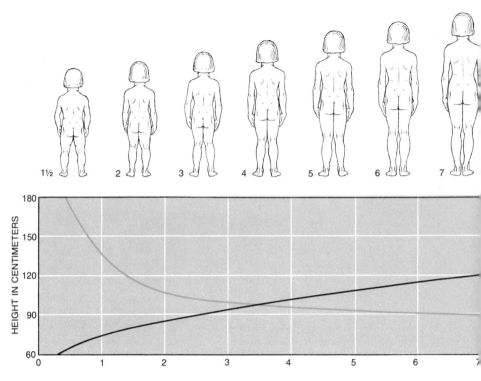

GIRL GROWING UP is shown at regular intervals from infancy to maturity (*top*). The figures show the change in the form of her body as well as her increase in height. The

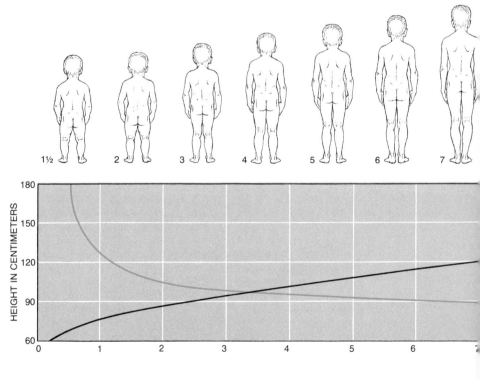

BOY GROWING UP is shown at the same age intervals as the girl. Again the height curve and velocity curve of his growth are below the figures that show the development of his

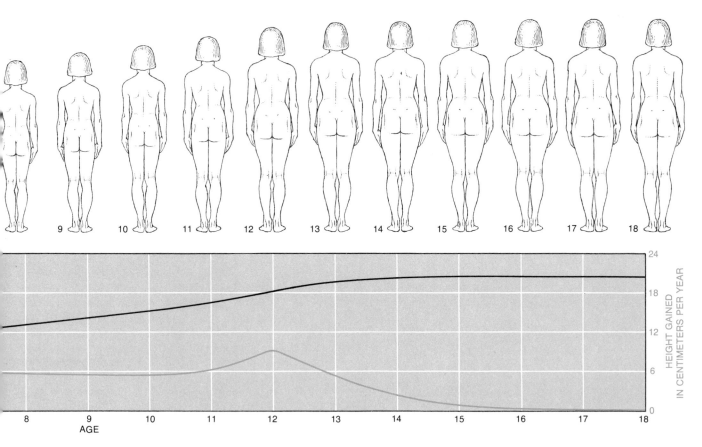

height curve (*black*) is an average for girls in North America and western Europe. Superposed on it is a curve for velocity of growth (*color*), which displays the increments of height gained from one age to the next. The sharp peak is the adolescent growth spurt.

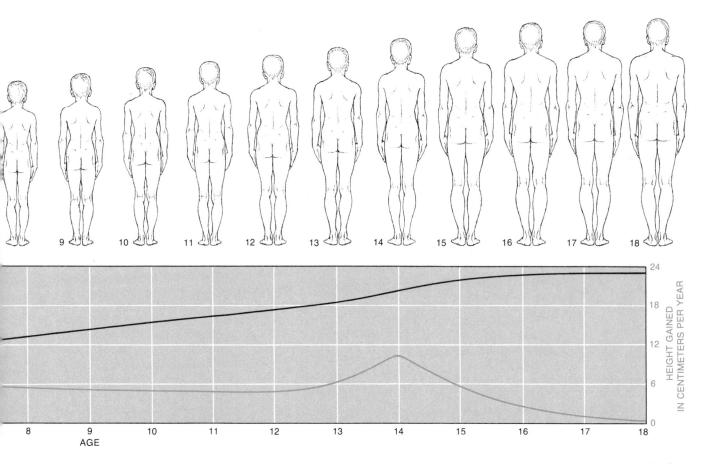

body. His adolescent growth spurt comes some two years later than the girl's. The human figures in both of these illustrations are based on photographs in the longitudinal-growth studies of Nancy Bayley and Leona Bayer of the University of California at Berkeley.

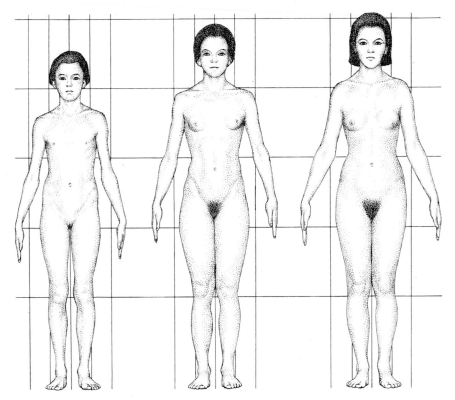

THREE GIRLS, all with the chronological age of 12.75 years, differed dramatically in development according to whether the particular girl had not yet reached puberty (*left*), was part of the way through it (*middle*) or had finished her development (*right*). This range of variation is completely normal. This drawing and the one below are based on photographs made by author and his colleagues at Institute of Child Health of University of London.

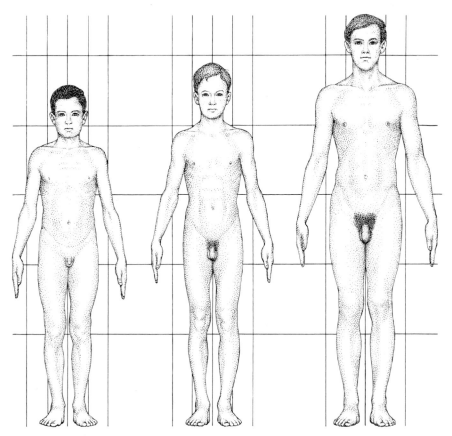

THREE BOYS, all of the chronological age of 14.75 years, showed a similar variation in the range of their development. As is indicated in the charts on page 22, evidently some boys have entirely finished their growth and sexual maturation before others even begin theirs.

tiates as female, that is, as an organ that will mediate the endocrinological functions of the female's sexual cycle. The same is probably true in man, with the sensitive period coming in the fourth month of fetal life.

Other sex differences develop gradually during the entire course of childhood growth. From birth onward males have larger forearms than females with respect to the length of their upper arms or to total body height. The velocity of growth in the length of the male's forearm is always slightly greater than the velocity of growth in the female's.

At puberty some of the more distinct sex differences appear, and the majority of them result in immediate differences in behavior. At about the same time that the adolescent growth spurt is under way, the reproductive system of both the male and the female begins to mature. In boys the growth of the penis and the testes accelerates. In girls the breasts begin to develop. In both sexes the pubic hair first appears. Even though girls experience their adolescent growth spurt two years earlier than boys, the sexes are separated only by six months in the first changes of puberty. Menarche is a late event in female puberty and invariably comes after the peak of the growth spurt is over.

Just as there are large variations in the normal range of childhood heights at any particular age, there are wide individual differences in the rates at which children develop—in what has been called the tempo of growth. These differences are present at all ages but their effects are seen most dramatically at adolescence. For example, the range of ages for the beginning of penis growth in males is from 10.5 to 14.5 years, and the range of ages for the completion of that development is from 12.5 to 16.5 years. Evidently some boys have finished their growth before others have even begun.

The importance of this variation in individuals for educational practice is obvious enough, although how to deal with it is less so. Body-contact sports between boys who are early maturers with boys of the same age who are late maturers are scarcely to be recommended. The situation is complicated by the fact that ability in school work and formal examinations is significantly, although not closely, linked to body size and the degree of development. Thus examinations administered to a group of children purely on the basis of their chronological age, such as the 11-plus examination in Britain, tend to pick out more than the fair share of earlier maturers for future advancement without any evidence that

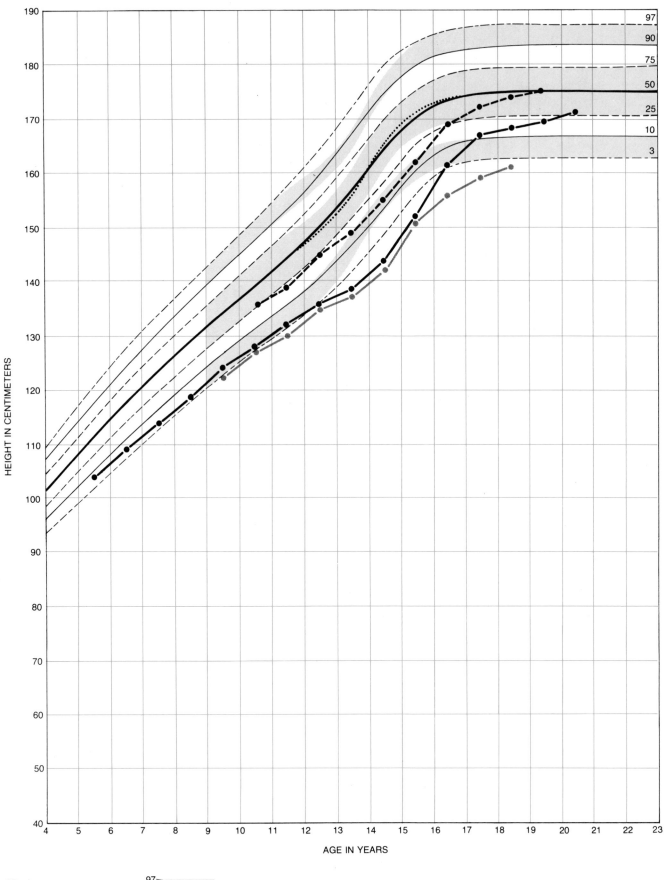

AGE IN YEARS

HEIGHT IN CENTIMETERS

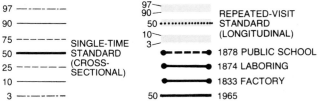

SECULAR TREND IN HEIGHT is shown by surveys of the height of English boys in the years 1833, 1874, 1878 and 1965. Data are reproduced on a standard growth chart. "Single-time standard (cross-sectional)" refers to the average result from cross-sectional surveys. "Repeated-visit standard (longitudinal)" refers to average result from longitudinal surveys. The numbers 97, 90, 75 and so on indicate percent of the male population shorter than a given height.

these would ultimately prove to be the brightest individuals in the group.

There is little doubt that being an early or a late maturer can have considerable and perhaps lasting effects on the individual's behavior. Perhaps boys are at more risk than girls, since the changes in their size and strength are greater. In one case two boys who were of equal height at age 11 differed three years later in height by 12 centimeters (five inches), by many kilograms of weight-lifting performance and by an entire dimension of sexual development. Part of the duty of teachers is to understand this aspect of biological variability, to recognize the late maturers and to reassure them that their ultimate status is not a jot different from that of the early maturers.

In the light of the variation in the tempo of growth, we need some measure of developmental age or physiological maturity that would be applicable throughout the entire period of growth. Numerous possible measurements have been tried, ranging from the number of teeth that have erupted to the amount of water in muscle cells. The various scales do not necessarily coincide; the most commonly used is bone age, or skeletal maturity. This measurement rests on the fact that the bones (in practice those of the hand and wrist) pass through the same developmental stages, independently of size, in all children. Therefore a scale can be constructed corresponding to how close the bone is to the adult appearance at any given time.

Bone age can be used to help in certain problems of educational guidance. The Royal School of Ballet in the United Kingdom insists that the height of dancers in its corps de ballet be within rather narrow limits. Its associated school takes in prospective dancers mostly at ages nine to 11. A considerable number of the children were found to end up as adults who were unacceptably tall or short. Their training had been wasted, their hopes dashed and their life disoriented. At the Institute of Child Health of the University of London, R. H. Whitehouse, W. A. Marshall and I developed a method for predicting adult height, derived originally from the work of Nancy Bayley of the University of California at Berkeley. Adult height is predicted by an equation involving present height, chronological age and bone age. The coefficients of the equations differ at age nine, 10 and so on; in puberty the importance of the bone-age coefficient increases and that of the chronological-age coefficient decreases. Thus for a 12-year-old girl one has a measure of whether she is advanced and nearing the end of her growth period or whether she is delayed and has much more growth to come.

The predictions are moderately successful. The great majority of the children are within five centimeters (two inches) of the actual height attained. We thus give the prediction in the form of a 10-centimeter band of adult height. If part of this band overlaps the required band for dancers, well and good; if it does not, the child is told of her limited chances for a dancing career. We are seeking ways of making the prediction better. Allowance for parental height improves it slightly, but the chief errors seem to come from our being unable to predict how large the adolescent spurt will be. The amount of height added in the spurt is largely independent of preadolescent growth. Very likely it has a separate genetic control.

The rate of growth at any age is clearly the outcome of the interaction of genetic and environmental factors. The child inherits possible patterns of growth from his parents. The environment, however, dictates which (if any) of the patterns will become actual. In an environ-

SEQUENCE OF EVENTS OF PUBERTY IN GIRLS at various ages is diagrammed for the average child. The hump in the bar labeled "Height spurt" represents the peak velocity of the spurt. The bars represent the beginning and completion of the events of puberty. Although the adolescent growth spurt for girls typically begins at age 10.5 and ends at age 14, it can start as early as age 9.5 and end as late as age 15. Similarly, menarche (the onset of menstruation) can come at any time between the ages of 10 and 16.5 and tends to be a late event of puberty. Some girls begin to show breast development as early as age eight and have completed it by age 13; others may not begin it until age 13 and complete it at age 18. First pubic hair appears after the beginning of breast development in two-thirds of all girls.

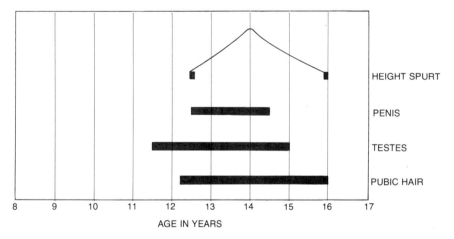

SEQUENCE OF EVENTS OF PUBERTY IN BOYS is also shown at various ages for the average child. The adolescent growth spurt of boys can begin as early as age 10.5 or as late as age 16 and can end anywhere from age 13.5 to age 17.5. Elongation of the penis can begin from age 10.5 to 14.5 and can end from age 12.5 to 16.5. Growth of the testes can begin as early as age 9.5 or as late as age 13.5 and end at any time between the ages of 13.5 and 17.

H — Phe —Pro — Thr — Ile — Pro — Leu — Ser — Arg — Leu — Phe — Asp —Asn —Ala — Met — Leu — Arg — Ala — His — Arg — Leu —
1   5   10   15   20

Gln — Glu — Lys — Pro — Ile — Tyr — Ala — Glu — Glu — Phe — Glu — Gln — Tyr — Thr — Asp —Phe —Ala — Leu —Gln — His —
40   35   30   25

Lys — Tyr — Ser — Phe —Leu —Gln — Asn —Pro — Gln — Thr — Ser — Leu — Cys — Phe — Ser — Glu — Ser — Ile — Pro — Thr —
45   50   55   60

Leu —Ser — Ile — Arg — Leu —Leu — Gln — Leu — Asn —Ser — Lys — Gln — Gln — Thr — Glu — Glu — Arg — Asn —Ser — Pro —
80   75   70   65

Leu —Leu —Ile — Gln — Ser — Trp — Leu —Glu — Pro — Val — Gln — Phe —Leu — Arg — Ser — Val — Phe —Ala — Asn —Ser —
85   90   95   100

Gly — Glu — Glu — Leu — Asp —Lys — Leu — Leu — Asp —Tyr — Val — Asp —Ser — Asn —Ser — Ala — Gly — Tyr — Val — Leu —
120   115   110   105

Ile — Gln — Thr — Leu —Met — Gly — Arg — Leu —Glu — Asp — Gly — Ser — Pro — Arg — Thr — Gly — Gln — Ile — Phe —Lys —
125   130   135   140

Tyr — Asn —Lys —Leu —Leu —Ala — Asp —Asp —Asn —His — Ser — Asn —Thr — Asp —Phe —Lys — Ser — Tyr — Thr — Gln —
160   155   150   145

Gly — Leu —Leu —Tyr — Cys —Phe —Arg — Lys — Asp —Met — Asp —Lys — Val — Glu — Thr — Phe — Leu — Arg — Ile — Val —
165   170   175   180

OH — Phe — Gly — Cys —Ser — Gly — Glu — Val — Ser — Arg — Cys —Gln —
190   185

Ala	ALANINE	Gly	GLYCINE
Arg	ARGININE	His	HISTIDINE
Asn	ASPARAGINE	Ile	ISOLEUCINE
Asp	ASPARTIC ACID	Leu	LEUCINE
Cys	CYSTINE	Lys	LYSINE
Gln	GLUTAMINE	Met	METHIONINE
Glu	GLUTAMIC ACID	Phe	PHENYLALANINE
Pro	PROLINE		
Ser	SERINE		
Thr	THREONINE		
Trp	TRYPTOPHAN		
Tyr	TYROSINE		
Val	VALINE		

HUMAN GROWTH HORMONE, also called somatotrophin, is a protein consisting of a chain of 191 amino acid units. The sequence of the amino acid units was presented in 1966 by Choh Hao Li of the University of California at Berkeley and was later modified by Hugh Niall of the Massachusetts General Hospital. Somatotrophin, acting with other hormones, regulates the normal growth of children. Lines joining two pairs of cystine (*Cys*) units represent disulfide bonds. Growth-hormone molecule is folded in such a way that paired cystine units are adjacent to each other.

ment where nutrition is always adequate, where the parents are caring and where social factors are adequate it is the genes that largely determine differences between members of the population in growth and in adult physique. In an environment that is suboptimal and perhaps changes from time to time, as in the periodic famines characteristic of much of the world, differences between members of the population reflect the social history of the individuals as much as their genetic endowment.

The genetic-environment interaction need not be additive. A child whose genes enable him to grow very well in an optimal environment may be less able to do so under poor circumstances than a child who in the good environment was smaller than he. Such differences in the degree to which growth can be regulated probably themselves depend largely on genetic factors. Girls are on the average better able to cope with environmental changes than boys, and their growth is less affected by such adverse factors as atomic radiation or poor nutrition. The same holds true in at least some other mammalian species.

The shape of the body is under closer genetic control than size. Identical twins may be so nearly the same in shape that they cannot be distinguished, yet one may be larger in absolute dimensions, usually from the time of birth. Japanese reared in California grew to be larger than Japanese in the then poorer nutritional circumstances of Japan, but their characteristic facial and trunk-limb proportions did not change. It seems that between blacks and whites in the U.S. and Jamaica there is very little difference in height when the circumstances of the two groups can be matched, but differences in the two groups' body proportions remain, American blacks having longer legs and arms and slenderer hips than American whites. Similar genetically controlled differences in proportion are observed between, for example, the Tutsi and Hutu, two African populations living side by side in Rwanda.

Since growth is so sensitive to malnutrition and other environmental upsets, surveys of the growth of children are an essential part of any country's monitoring of its social and nutritional status. When such surveys are carried out with the proper attention to sampling, the proper training of the measurers and the proper recording of the relevant social data, they can clearly indicate the factors causing childhood disadvantage. These factors usually include the number of siblings in the family, the occupation and income of the parents and the physical geography of the region: whether it is mountainous or low-lying, hot or cold.

Complications arise in countries where the population is not genetically homogeneous, or where social class and ethnic origin are related. Even in these cases, however, standards can be set for each ethnic group. In my opinion standards for developing countries should not be constructed from a random sample of the entire population, as standards in well-nourished countries are. In countries that are subject to general malnutrition, standards should be based on a sample of the population that is environmentally faring the best, since these individuals represent the currently attainable range of desired norms for the population as a whole.

As the environmental and social conditions of a country improve, the children grow up faster and reach a greater final size. The variation between individuals of different social classes becomes less. This process is termed the secular trend of growth. In Europe and North America the process has been going on continuously for about 100 years. The first survey of a population in the United Kingdom was the measurement of the height of boys working in factories in 1833. The results of this early survey can be compared with the results of a survey of boys of the working classes and of the upper middle classes carried out from 1874 through 1878 and with the results of a modern survey of London boys in 1965.

The effect of the environment on the boys' rate of maturation is considerably greater than its effect on the boys' final size. In the 19th century working-class boys went on growing far into their middle twenties and thus eventually made up for some of their earlier deficit. Victor Oppers of the Amsterdam department of health has estimated that the secular trend of final adult size in the Netherlands was zero between 1820 and 1860. Between 1860 and 1960, however, it was one centimeter per decade. In other words, the average adult in 1960 was 10 centimeters (four inches) taller than his counterpart of a century ago.

There has also been a downward secular trend in the age of menarche. In some countries where the statistics are adequate there was a trend of three to four months per decade from 1840 to 1960. There are indications that the trend has ceased in some populations, such as in Oslo, in London and in the upper social classes in the U.S. In others, however, it is still active. The trend of increasing height has also nearly ceased in American and British populations that are economically well off.

Although the reasons for secular trends are not fully understood, it seems likely that better nutrition, particularly in infancy, is chiefly responsible. In many countries today, however, there is a danger that children are being overfed. Childhood obesity is becoming common, particularly where children are fed from bottles and are given solid food very early instead of (or in addition to) breast-feeding. In these circumstances surveys of growth are still highly important, but measurements of skin folds, which are an indication of the amount of subcutaneous fat, have to be added to measurements of height and weight.

The mechanisms through which growth is genetically controlled are obscure. Indeed, the reason one child grows faster and to a greater adult height than another is quite unknown. All we can say at present is that certain hormones are essential for normal growth. Among them are the pituitary growth hormone, the thyroid hormone, insulin and the gonadotropic and sex hormones.

Lack of growth hormone causes a particular form of dwarfism. (The term is never used in the clinic, since it tends to conjure up associations with elves and demons. We refer to these children as suffering from short stature.) Such children are normal at birth but fail to grow adequately in length thereafter (although they may at first apparently gain weight normally, due to the accumulation of excessive fat). Human growth hormone, extracted from the pituitary gland of cadavers, is now available for the treatment of short stature due to growth-hormone deficiency. Such treatment results in a period of supernormal growth, which has been called "catch up" growth. Catch-up growth is characteristic of all children whose normal development has been retarded (for example by malnutrition) and then resumes when the retarding factor is removed. Growth-hormone-deficient children require growth hormone continuously throughout childhood and adolescence in order to attain normal adult stature.

The condition seems to be due to a malfunction of the hypothalamus rather than of the pituitary gland itself. Like all pituitary hormones, growth hormone is controlled by a specific releasing hormone secreted by the cells of the hypothalamus. The deficiency may be simply in the amount of growth hormone, or it may extend to the release of other pituitary hormones as well. The deficiency occurs in families. Some 15 percent of the siblings of these patients and 1 to 2 percent of the parents also lack growth hormone.

Growth hormone seems to completely restore the capacity of these children to grow. If it is given early enough, the child catches up totally and ends up at, or very near, his genetically programmed curve. Interestingly enough, giving excess growth hormone produces no excess growth. By the same token giving growth hormone to normal children, who have their own supply, fails to increase their size.

Growth hormone does not act directly on growing cartilage. It causes the liver to secrete another hormone: somatomedin. The somatomedin molecule is much smaller than the growth hormone molecule, but its structure is not yet known. Whether or not somatomedin could be administered to cause normal small children to grow to be normal large children is not known. The possibility, however, seems unlikely. The ultimate control of the size of a child probably lies in the number of cartilage cells he has and their responsiveness to the various hormones.

In certain forms of dwarfism it is these cartilage cells that are at fault. The best-known of these growth disorders is called achondroplasia. Here the defect is localized chiefly in the bones of the upper arm and the thigh. Achondroplasia is an inherited disorder; a single dominant gene is responsible.

In some children the secretion of the growth-hormone releaser may be switched off as a result of psychosocial upset. Such children resemble others who have a deficiency of growth hormone, except that they usually also have a history of psychiatric disturbance and abnormal behavior. Furthermore, when these children are removed from their stressful surroundings, their growth hormone switches on again and they show typical catch-up growth. This phenomenon was first described under the name of deprivation dwarfism by Lytt I. Gardner of the Upstate Medical Center of the State University of New York and by Robert M. Blizzard and his colleagues at the Johns Hopkins Hospital [see "Deprivation Dwarfism," by Lytt I. Gardner; SCIENTIFIC AMERICAN, July, 1972]. It is now more usually called psychosocial short stature, since "deprivation" does not always adequately describe the social process that gives rise to it.

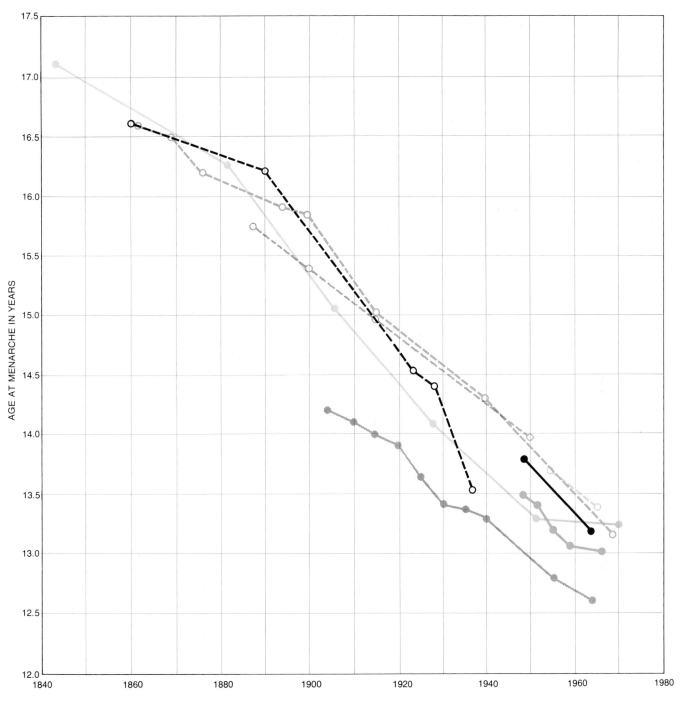

AGE OF MENARCHE in the U.S. and seven countries of western Europe has declined greatly from what it was 120 years ago. For example, in the mid-1840's an average Norwegian girl began menstruating at 17; today she is just over 13. The downward trend appears to be leveling off in the case of some countries. Trend is probably chiefly due to advances in nutrition over the past century.

In addition to growth hormone the sex hormones are required for normal growth in prenatal life and at puberty, and perhaps also in the years before puberty. They are present in small quantities in the blood throughout growth, but the quantities increase greatly at puberty. Testosterone is responsible for much of the adolescent spurt in boys, although growth hormone is still necessary; the growth rate of boys deficient in growth hormone is greater when they are given growth hormone plus testosterone than when they are given either hormone alone. The adolescent growth spurt in girls, however, seems to be caused by growth hormone plus androgenic hormones from the adrenal gland. The female sex hormone (estrogen) does not give rise to growth, except growth of the breasts and of the reproductive tract.

Much about the mechanism of growth and maturation still remains obscure.

Our lack of specific information does not prevent the use of growth rates as a guide for improving the health of populations, nor does it impair the importance of a knowledge of variation in growth rates, both between and within the sexes. Nevertheless, human biologists would dearly like to know the movement of each of the particular hormonal shuttles that weave the complex and unique patterns that constitute an individual's growing up.

III

Getting Old

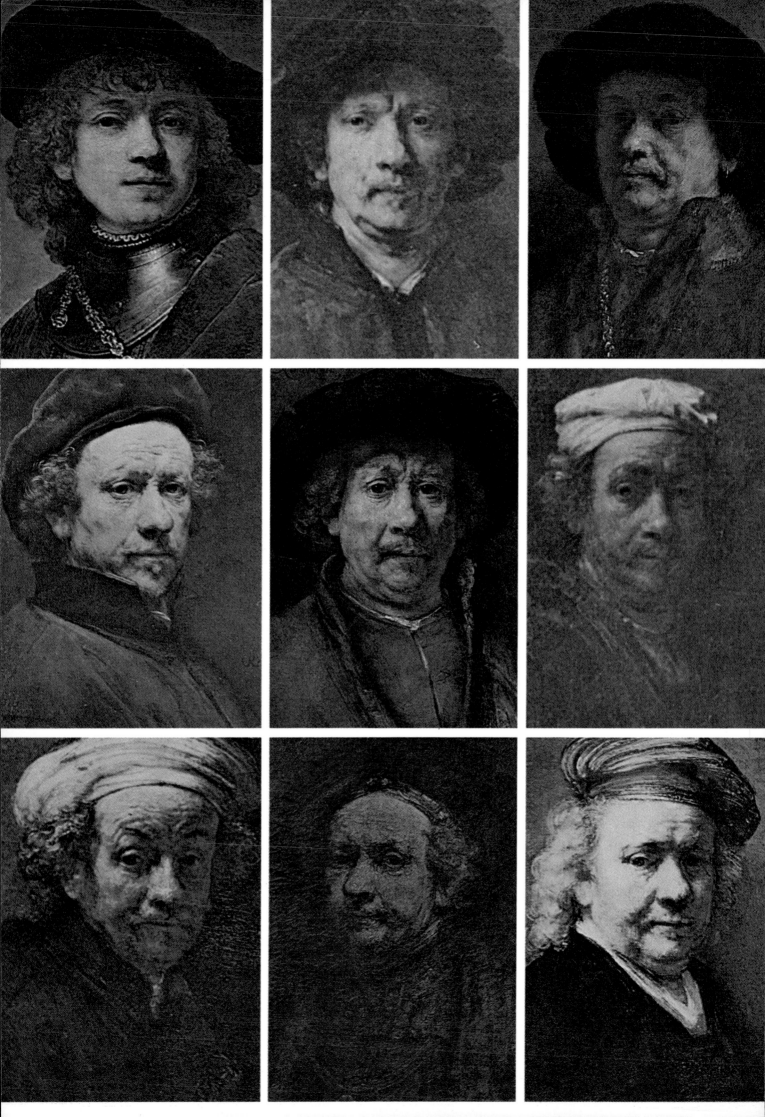

Getting Old

ALEXANDER LEAF

Everyone ages, but some seem to age less quickly than others. In search of clues to the phenomenon the author visits three communities where vigorous oldsters are remarkably numerous

"The patient, Mr. X, is 81 years old. A resident of the Dunhill Nursing Home, he has had two strokes, the first three years ago and the second a year ago. Since the last stroke he has been bedridden, incontinent and senile. He no longer recognizes members of his own family. For the past two months he has been eating poorly and failing generally. He was brought in last night by ambulance to our Emergency Service, where we found pulmonary congestion from a failing arteriosclerotic heart and pneumonia. Treatment was started with diuretics and digitalis for his congestive heart failure and high doses of penicillin for his pneumonia. This morning his fever is gone and he is breathing quietly."

I listen to this familiar story related by my intern at the Massachusetts General Hospital and mentally fill in the remainder of the picture. Sometimes the patient is 65, sometimes 70 or 90. Sometimes there is an underlying cancer. Usually, however, cardiovascular or respiratory problems dominate the clinical situation but are superimposed on a substrate of debility, wasting and senility. In the past pneumonia usually terminated such stories with some degree of dignity. Today modern medicine, with its antibiotics, intravenous infusions, cardiac

pacemakers, respirators, diuretics and the like can often resolve the immediate problem (pneumonia and congestive heart failure in this instance) and return the patient to his nursing home again.

In a large metropolitan teaching hospital some 40 percent of the medical (as opposed to surgical) beds are occupied by patients over 65, many of them in a condition similar to Mr. X's. More than 20 million citizens are 65 or older in the U.S. today. They are the major reservoir of illness and medical needs. When I chose a career in medicine 35 years ago, I did so with the conviction that regardless of my eventual specialization my work would promote health and relieve human suffering. Today I contemplate Mr. X and wonder if my initial conviction was right. Of course, medicine does more than treat the Mr. X's, but are we doing the best we can for contemporary society? The proportion of the population over 65 is between 10 and 11 percent now and will come close to 15 percent in the next few decades. What is medicine doing about it? Are we applying our resources wisely? Should we devote proportionately more of our efforts to trying to learn how we can prevent the infirmities of old age?

In the U.S. in 1969 the life expectancy at birth for white males was 67.8 years

and for white females 75.1 years. That is some 23 years longer than life expectancy was in 1900. However, an adult who had reached 65 at the turn of the century could expect to live another 13 years and an adult who reaches 65 today can expect to live another 15 years, or only two years longer than in 1900. The seemingly large increase in life expectancy at birth actually reflects the great reduction in infant mortality. Little progress has been made in controlling the major causes of death in adults: heart disease, cancer and stroke. Accidents, of which nearly half are caused by motor vehicles, are a fourth major cause of adult deaths.

At the Ninth International Congress of Gerontology in July, 1972, M. Vacek of Czechoslovakia discussed the increase in mean age and the rising proportion of old people in the population. He pointed out the fact that the rise in the number of people over 65 toward 15 percent in the populations of stable, industrial countries could be attributed to a falling birthrate. When at the conclusion of his remarks someone in the audience timidly asked if the achievements of the medical sciences had played a role in the rise in mean age, he responded that indeed they had, but that the simultaneous deterioration of the environment had canceled out any positive effect from medicine.

Mere length of life, however, may be a poor concern on which to focus. Most would agree that the quality of life, rather than its duration, should be the prime issue. The active life, so warmly espoused by Theodore Roosevelt, has been the American model. If one can extend the period of productive activity as did Verdi and Churchill, so much the better.

Most students of the field would agree

NINE REMBRANDT SELF-PORTRAITS, painted between the ages of 27 or 28 and 63, document the progress of aging in the case of a generally prosperous Dutch burgher of the mid-17th century. The painter was born in July, 1606, and died in October, 1669. His self-portrait of 1633 or 1634 (*top left on opposite page*) is now in the Uffizi Gallery in Florence. Next (*top center*) is his self-portrait of 1652, when he was 46 years old. This is one of three portraits reproduced here that are in the Kunsthistorisches Museum in Vienna. Next (*top right*) is a portrait at age 49, also in Vienna. The second row begins (*left*) with a portrait in the National Gallery of Scotland in Edinburgh, painted at the age of 51. Next is the third of the Vienna paintings, which may show Rembrandt one year older (*center*). At the right is his portrait at age 54, now in the Louvre. The bottom row begins (*left*) with a portrait at age 55, now in the Rijksmuseum in Amsterdam. The next portrait (*center*) may have been painted in 1664 when Rembrandt was 58; it is also in the Uffizi. The last portrait (*right*) Rembrandt painted in the year of his death; it is at the Mauritshuis in The Hague.

with the statement of Frédéric Verzár, the Swiss dean of gerontologists. "Old age is not an illness," says Verzár. "It is a continuation of life with decreasing capacities for adaptation." The main crippler and killer, arteriosclerosis, is not a necessary accompaniment of aging but a disease state that increases in incidence with age; the same is true of cancer. If we could prevent arteriosclerosis, hypertension and cancer, the life-span could be pushed back closer to the biological limit, if such a limit in fact exists.

In order to observe aged individuals who are free of debilitating illness I recently visited three remote parts of the world where the existence of such individuals was rumored. These were the village of Vilcabamba in Ecuador, the small principality of Hunza in West Pakistan and the highlands of Georgia in the Soviet Caucasus.

A census of Vilcabamba taken in 1971 by Ecuador's National Institute of Statistics recorded a total population of 819 in this remote Andean village. Nine of the 819 were over 100 years old. The proportion of the population in this small village over 60 is 16.4 percent, as contrasted with a figure of 6.4 percent for rural Ecuador in general. The valley that shelters Vilcabamba is at an altitude of some 4,500 feet. Its vegetation appears quite lush. The people live by farming, but the methods are so primitive that only a bare subsistence is extracted from the land.

A team of physicians and scientists from Quito under the direction of Miguel

Salvador has been studying this unique population. Guillermo Vela of the University of Quito, the nutritionist in the group, finds that the average daily caloric intake of an elderly Vilcabamba adult is 1,200 calories. Protein provided 35 to 38 grams and fat only 12 to 19 grams; 200 to 250 grams of carbohydrate completed the diet. The contribution of animal protein and animal fat to the diet is very low.

The villagers of Vilcabamba, like most inhabitants of underdeveloped countries, live without benefit of modern sanitation, cleanliness and medical care. Cleanliness is evidently not a prerequisite for longevity. A small river skirts the village and provides water for drinking, washing and bathing. When we asked various villagers how long it had been since they had last bathed, the responses showed that many had not done so for two years. (The record was 10 years.) The villagers live in mud huts with dirt floors; chickens and pigs share their quarters. As one might expect in such surroundings, infant mortality is high, but so is the proportion of aged individuals. By extrapolation it stands at 1,100 per 100,000, compared with three per 100,000 in the U.S. Statistically, of course, such an extrapolation from so small a number is unwarranted; nonetheless, it shows how unusual the age distribution is in this little village.

The old people of Vilcabamba all appeared to be of European rather than Indian descent. We were able to validate the reported ages of almost all the elderly individuals from baptismal records

kept in the local Catholic church. Miguel Carpio, aged 121, was the oldest person in the village when we were there. José Toledo's picture has appeared in newspapers around the world with captions that have proclaimed his extreme old age; actually he is only 109. All the old people were born locally, so that what is sometimes called the Miami Beach phenomenon, that is, an ingathering of the elderly, cannot account for the age distribution.

Both tobacco and sugarcane are grown in the valley, and a local rum drink, *zuhmir*, is produced. We did not, however, witness any drunkenness, and although most villagers smoke, there is disagreement among visiting physicians about how many of them inhale. The villagers work hard to scratch a livelihood from the soil, and the mountainous terrain demands continuous and vigorous physical activity. These circumstances are hardly unique to Vilcabamba, and one leaves this Andean valley with the strong suspicion that genetic factors must be playing an important role in the longevity of this small enclave of elderly people of European stock.

The impression that genetic factors are important in longevity was reinforced by what we saw in Hunza. This small independent state is ruled over by a hereditary line of leaders known as Mirs. In 1891 the Mir of that day surrendered control over defense, communications and foreign affairs to the British when they conquered his country. In 1948, after the partition of Pakistan and India,

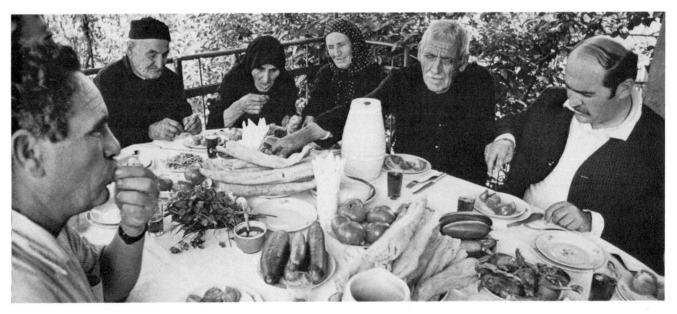

IN SOVIET GEORGIA, one of three widely separated parts of the world visited by the author, a 105-year-old man has the place of honor (*at head of table, left*) at a party held near the village of Gurjanni. The centenarian was the oldest guest but the man and the two women on his left are all over 80. The average diet of those over 80 in the Caucasus is relatively rich in proteins (70 to 80 grams a day) and fats (40 to 60 grams), but the daily caloric intake, 1,700 to 1,900 calories, is barely half the U.S. average.

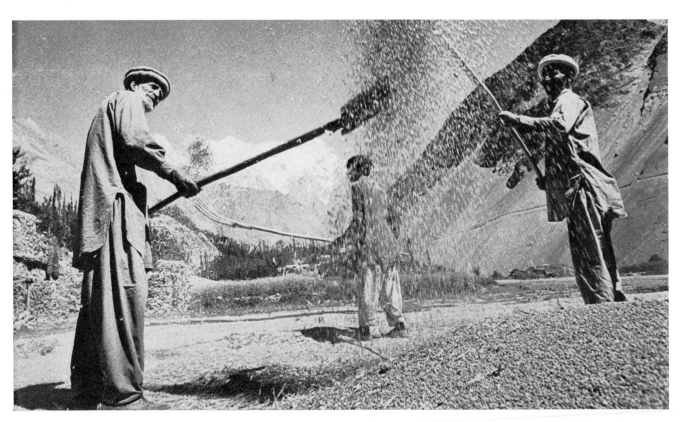

ON THE PAKISTAN FRONTIER old men of the principality of Hunza, another area visited by the author, winnow threshed wheat in a mountain village. Ibriham Shah (*right*) professes to be 80 years old but Mohd Ghraib (*left*) says he is only 75. Both vigorous work and a low-calorie diet are factors in the fitness of Hunza elders. An adult male's daily diet includes 50 grams of proteins, 36 grams of fats and 354 grams of carbohydrate. This combination provides a somewhat higher daily total than in the Caucasus: 1,923 calories.

the present Mir yielded the same right to Pakistan. Hunza is hidden among the towering peaks of the Karakorum Range on Pakistan's border with China and Afghanistan and is one of the most inaccessible places on the earth. After a day's travel from Gilgit, first by jeep and then on foot from the point where a rockslide had cut the mountain road, we found ourselves in a valley surrounded on all sides by peaks more than 20,000 feet high, blocked at the far end by Mount Rokaposhi, which rises to 25,500 feet in snow-clad splendor.

The valley is arid, but a system of irrigation canals built over the past 800 years carries water from the high surrounding glaciers, converting the valley into a terraced garden. The inhabitants work their fields by primitive agricultural methods, and the harvests are not quite sufficient to prevent a period of real privation each winter. According to S. Maqsood Ali, a Pakistani nutritionist who has surveyed the diet of 55 adult males in Hunza, the daily diet averages 1,923 calories: 50 grams are protein, 36 grams fat and 354 grams carbohydrate. Meat and dairy products accounted for only 1 percent of the total. Land is too precious to be used to support dairy herds; the few animals that are kept by the people are killed for meat only dur-

ing the winter or on festive occasions.

As in Vilcabamba, everyone in Hunza works hard to wrest a living from the rocky hills. One sees an unusual number of vigorous people who, although elderly in appearance, agilely climb up and down the steep slopes of the valley. Their language is an unwritten one, so that no documentary records of birth dates are available. In religion the Hunzakuts are Ismaili Moslems, followers of the Agha Khan. Their education is quite limited. Thus, although a number of nonscientific accounts have attributed remarkable longevity and robust health to these people, no documentation substantiates the reports.

Unfortunately there is no known means of distinguishing chronological age from physiological age in humans. When we asked elderly Hunzakuts how old they were and what they remembered of the British invasion of their country in 1891, their answers did little to validate their supposed age. If, however, they are as old as both they and their Mir, a well-educated and worldly man, maintain, then there are a remarkable number of aged but lean and fit-looking Hunzakuts who can climb the steep slopes of their valley with far greater ease than we could. Putatively the oldest citizen was one Tulah Beg,

who said he was 110; the next oldest, also a male, said he was 105.

In addition to their low-calorie diet, which is also low in animal fats, and their intense physical activity, the Hunzakuts have a record of genetic isolation that must be nearly unique. Now, there do not seem to be "good" genes that favor longevity but only "bad" genes that increase the probability of acquiring a fatal illness. One may therefore speculate that a small number of individuals, singularly lacking such "bad" genes, settled this mountain valley centuries ago and that their isolation has prevented a subsequent admixture with "bad" genes. This, of course, is mere speculation.

The possible role of genetic factors in longevity seemed of less importance in the Caucasus. In Abkhasia on the shores of the Black Sea and in the adjoining Caucasus one encounters many people over 100 who are not only Georgian but also Russian, Jewish, Armenian and Turkish. The Caucasus is a land bridge that has been traveled for centuries by conquerors from both the east and the west, and its population can scarcely have maintained any significant degree of genetic isolation. At the same time, when one speaks to the numerous

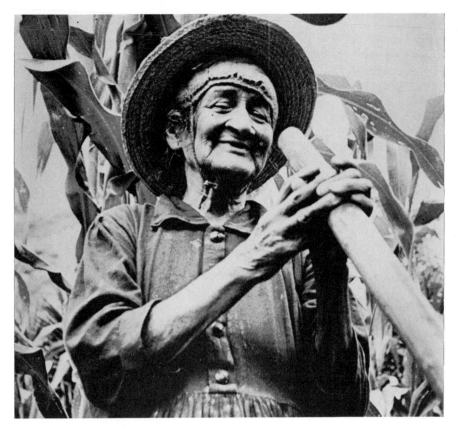

IN THE ANDES OF ECUADOR an 85-year-old woman of the village of Vilcabamba works in a cornfield, continuing to contribute to the economic welfare of the community at an age when many women no longer work. Of the areas visited by the author, Vilcabamba afforded the elderly the most sparse diet. The daily intake was less than 40 grams of proteins, 20 grams of fats and 250 grams of carbohydrate for a total intake of 1,200 calories.

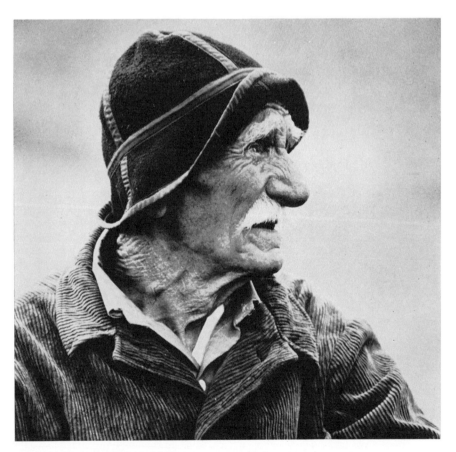

BLACK SEA VILLAGER from the coast near Sukhumi is over 100 years old. To live to be 100 or older in the Caucasus gains one a kind of elder statesman's place in local society.

centenarians in the area, one invariably discovers that each of them has parents or siblings who have similarly attained great age. The genetic aspect of longevity therefore cannot be entirely dismissed.

In contrast to the isolated valleys of Vilcabamba and Hunza, the Caucasus is an extensive area that includes three Soviet republics: Georgia, Azerbaijan and Armenia. The climate varies from the humid and subtropical (as at Sukhumi on the Black Sea, with an annual rainfall of 1,100 to 1,400 millimeters) to drier continental conditions, marked by extremes of summer heat and winter cold. The population extends from sea-level settlements along the Black and Caspian seas to mountain villages at altitudes of 1,000 to 1,500 meters. More old people are found in the mountainous regions than at sea level, and the incidence of atherosclerosis among those who live in the mountains is only half that in the sea-level villages. G. Z. Pitzkhelauri, head of the Gerontological Center in the Republic of Georgia, told me that the 1970 census placed the number of centenarians for the entire Caucasus at between 4,500 and 5,000. Of these, 1,844, or an average of 39 per 100,000, live in Georgia. In Azerbaijan there are 2,500 more, or 63 per 100,000. Perhaps of more pertinence to my study was the record of activity among the elderly of the Caucasus. Of 15,000 individuals over 80 whose records were kept by Pitzkhelauri, more than 70 percent continue to lead very active lives. Sixty percent of them were still working on state or collective farms.

I returned from my three surveys convinced that a vigorous, active life involving physical activity (sexual activity included) was possible for at least 100 years and in some instances for even longer.

Longevity is clearly a multifactorial matter. First are the genetic factors; all who have studied longevity are convinced of their importance. It is generally accepted that the offspring of long-lived parents live longer than others. Yet a long life extends beyond the period of fertility, at least in women, so that length of life can have no direct evolutionary advantage. It has been suggested that living organisms are like clocks: their life-span ends when the initial endowment of energy is expended, just as the clock stops when its spring becomes unwound. L. V. Heilbrunn estimated in the 1900's that the heart of a mouse, which beats 520 to 780 times per minute, would contract 1.11 billion times during the 3.5 years of the mouse's normal life-span. The heart of an elephant, which beats 25 to 28 times per minute, would have beaten 1.021 billion times during the elephant's normal life-span of 70 years. The similarity between these two figures seems to suggest some initial equal potential that is gradually dissipated over the animal's life-span. Such calculations, however, are probably more entertaining than explanatory of longevity.

As I have mentioned, genes evidently influence longevity only in a negative way by predisposing the organism to specific fatal diseases. Alex Comfort of University College London has pointed out the possible role of heterosis, or "hybrid vigor." The crossbreeding of two inbred strains—each with limited growth, size, resistance to disease and longevity—can improve these characteristics in the progeny. This vigor has been manifested in a wide variety of species, both plant and animal, but its significance in human longevity is not known.

Next are the factors associated with nutrition. Since we are composed of what we eat and drink, it is not surprising that students of longevity have emphasized the importance of dietary factors. Indeed, the only demonstrable means of extending the life-span of an experimental animal has been the manipulation of diet. The classic studies of Clive M. McCay of Cornell University in the 1930's showed that the life-span of albino rats could be increased as much as 40 percent by the restriction of caloric intake early in life. Rats fed a diet otherwise balanced but deficient in calories showed delayed growth and maturation until the caloric intake was increased. At the same time their life-span was extended. The significance of these experiments with respect to human longevity is not known, but they raise questions about the current tendency to overfeed children.

The role of specific dietary factors in promoting longevity remains unsettled. When the old people we visited were asked to what they attributed their long life, credit was usually given to the local alcoholic beverage, but this response generally came from the more vocal and chauvinistic males. Much publicity is given today to the possible role of animal fats in the development of arteriosclerosis. Saturated fatty acids and cholesterol have also been suggested as the causal agents of coronary atherosclerosis. Since the atheromas themselves—the deposits that narrow and occlude the blood vessels of the heart, the brain and other organs—contain cholesterol, the suspicion

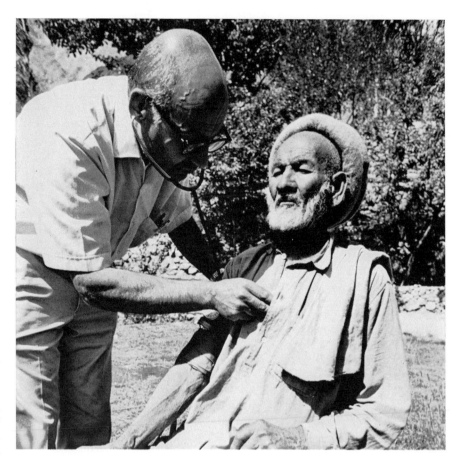

ELDER OF HUNZA is examined by the author. A resident of the village of Mominabad, the man professed to be 110 years old. Birth records are not kept in Hunza, however, and evidence supporting his claim and other Hunza elders' claims of extreme age did not exist.

of complicity comes easily. It is also well documented that the level of cholesterol in the blood serum has a positive prognostic relation to the likelihood of heart attacks.

Since the diet of affluent societies has a high content of animal fats, which are rich in cholesterol and saturated fatty acids, the suspicion further arises that these dietary constituents are contributing to the increase in the number of heart attacks affecting young adult males. The marked individual variability in tolerance to the quantity of fat and cholesterol in the diet, however, makes it difficult to ascribe prime importance to this single factor. We have seen that in both Vilcabamba and Hunza the diet was not only low in calories but also low in animal fats. In the Caucasus an active dairy economy allows cheese and milk products to be served with every meal. Perhaps it is significant that in this area the cheese is low in fat content and the total fat intake is only some 40 to 60 grams per day. This level is in sharp contrast to figures from a recent U.S. Department of Agriculture report stating that the average daily fat intake for Americans of all ages is 157 grams. The best-informed medical opinion today

generally agrees that the Americans' average daily intake of 3,300 calories, including substantial quantities of fat, is excessive and conducive neither to optimal health nor to longevity.

Let us now consider physical activity. There is increasing awareness that early heart disease is a price we are paying for our largely sedentary existence. In the three areas I visited physical fitness was an inevitable consequence of the active life led by the inhabitants. My initial speculation that their isolated lives protects them from the ravages of infectious diseases and from acquiring "bad" genes is probably incorrect. A simpler explanation for their fitness is that their mountainous terrain demands a high level of physical activity simply to get through the day.

A number of studies have examined the effects of physical activity on the incidence and severity of heart attacks among various sample populations. For example, among British postal workers it was found that those who delivered the mail had a lower incidence of heart attacks and, when attacks did occur, a lower mortality rate than their colleagues who worked at sedentary jobs. This same study also compared the relative incidence of heart attacks among London bus drivers and conductors. The conductors, who spent their working hours climbing up and down the double-deck buses collecting fares, had less heart trouble than the sedentary drivers. It has been reported recently that the weekend athlete who engages in vigorous physical activity is only one-third as prone to heart disease as his age-matched sedentary neighbor. It is well known that exercise increases the oxygenation of the blood and improves the circulation. Exercise will also improve the collateral circulation of blood to the heart muscle. When the exercises are carefully graded and performed under appropriate supervision, they are undoubtedly the best means of rehabilitating the heart muscle after a heart attack.

Exercise improves circulation to nearly all parts of the body. Circulation is increased to the brain as well as to the heart and skeletal muscles. Recently it has been asserted that improvement in the oxygen supply to the brain will actually improve thinking. In a resting sedentary individual, however, the blood supplied to the brain contains more oxygen than the brain is able to extract. It is difficult to explain how an added overabundance of a constituent that is normally not a rate-limiting factor in

cerebral function would enhance that function. It may nonetheless be that the sense of well-being that the exercising individual enjoys is likely to increase self-confidence and as a result improve both social and intellectual effectiveness.

Finally, physical activity helps to burn off excess calories and dispose of ingested fats. Exercise may thus counteract the deleterious effects of a diet that includes too many calories and too much fat. Indeed, it may well be one factor that helps to account for the great individual differences in tolerance for dietary factors.

Psychological factors must also be considered. It is characteristic of each of the areas I visited that the old people continue to be contributing, productive members of their society. The economy in all three areas is agrarian, there is no fixed retirement age and the elderly make themselves useful doing many necessary tasks around the farm or the home. Moreover, increased age is accompanied by increased social status. The old people, with their accumulated experience of life, are expected to be wise, and they respond accordingly. In Hunza the Mir rules his small state with the advice of a council of elders, who sit on the ground in a circle at his feet and help him with his decisions and pro-

nouncements. When we met Temur Tarba in the Caucasus just three weeks after his 100th birthday, it was clear from his manner that he was delighted to have at last "arrived." He proudly displayed his Hero of Labor medal, the highest civilian award of the U.S.S.R. He had won it only seven years earlier for his work in hybridizing corn. The cheerful centenarian still picked tea leaves, rode his horse and worked on a collective farm.

People who no longer have a necessary role to play in the social and economic life of their society generally deteriorate rapidly. The pattern of increasingly early retirement in our own society takes a heavy toll of our older citizens. They also find that their offspring generally have neither any room nor any use for them in their urban apartment. These are economic determinants that cannot be reversed in our culture today. Their devastating effect on the happiness and life-span of the elderly could be countered at least in part by educational programs to awaken other interests or avocations to which these people could turn with zest when their contribution to the industrial economy is no longer needed. The trend toward shorter working hours and earlier retirement makes the need for such education urgent. It seems a corruption of the very purpose of an economy that instead of freeing us from drudgery and need and allowing us to enjoy a better life, it holds us slaves to its dictates even though affluence is at hand.

In their remote farms and villages the old people I visited live oblivious to the pressures and strains of modern life. Such American controversies as the fighting in Southeast Asia, conflict in the Middle East, environmental pollution, the energy crisis and the like that fill our news media were unknown to them. Of course, most of the stresses and tensions to which mankind is subject arise from more personal social interactions, such as a quarrel with a spouse or misbehavior by an offspring. As a result it is impossible for any social group to entirely escape mental stress and tensions. Nonetheless, in societies that are less competitive and less aggressive even these personal stresses can be less exhausting than they are in our own. The old people I met abroad showed equanimity and optimism. In the Caucasus I asked Gabriel Chapnian, aged 117, what he thought of young people, of his government and of the state of the world in general. When he repeatedly responded "Fine, fine," I asked with some annoy-

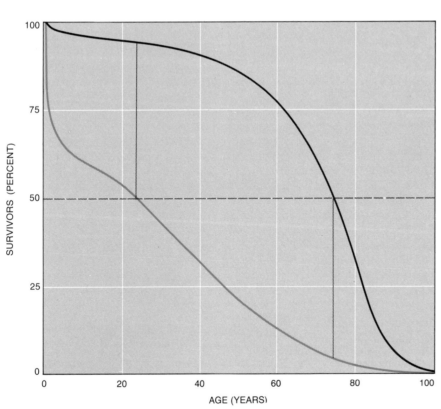

FEW LIVE TO GROW OLD in underdeveloped nations, whereas the opposite is true in the developed nations. For example, half of the women who died in India (*color*) from 1921 to 1930 were 24 or younger; only 5 percent of the women who died in New Zealand from 1934 to 1938 were that young. Half of the New Zealand women who died in the same period were 74 or older. In India only 5 percent of women's deaths were in this age group.

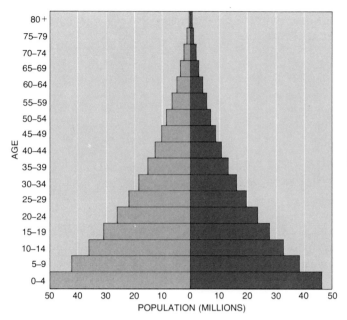

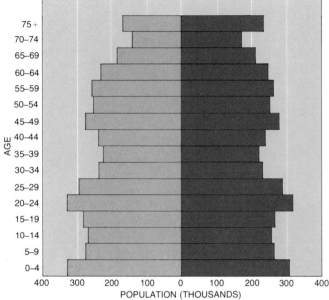

EXAGGERATED PYRAMID appears when the males (*left*) and females (*right*) of a population with a high growth rate are counted in ascending five-year steps. The graph shows the 1970 population of India; many more Indians are below the age of 20 than are above that age. In such an expanding population the elderly, although numerous, comprise a small percentage of the total.

UNEVEN COLUMN, rather than a pyramid, appears when the number of males (*left*) and females (*right*) in a slow-growing population are similarly displayed. The graph shows the population of Sweden in 1970; about as many Swedes are above the age of 35 as are below that age. In this population, noted for its low birthrate, the elderly comprise an increasingly large percentage of the total.

ance, "Isn't there anything today that disturbs you?" He replied cheerfully, "Oh yes, there are a number of things that are not the way I would want them to be, but since I can't change them I don't worry about them."

One cannot discuss the quality of life at advanced age without considering sexual activity. In most societies the combination of male boasting about sexual prowess and taboos against discussing the subject makes it difficult to collect reliable information about sexual activity in the elderly. Women's ovaries stop functioning at menopause, usually in the late 40's or early 50's, but this has little influence on the libido. Similarly, aging is associated with a gradual decrease in the number of cells in certain organs, including the male testes. The cells that produce sperm are the first to be affected, but later the cells that produce the male hormone testosterone may also diminish. in number and activity. Sexual potency in the male and libido in the female may nonetheless persist in advanced old age. Herman Brotman of the Department of Health, Education, and Welfare reports that each year there are some 3,500 marriages among the 20 million Americans over the age of 65, and that sexual activity is cited along with companionship as one reason for these late unions.

Research on aging is proceeding in two general directions. One aims at a better understanding of those disease states that, although they are not an integral part of the aging process, nevertheless increase in incidence with age and constitute the major cripplers of the aged. Here both arteriosclerosis and cancer are prominent. Knowledge of the causes and prevention of these diseases is still very limited, and much more work is necessary before there can be sufficient understanding to allow prevention of either. If both arteriosclerosis and cancer could be prevented, it should be possible to extend man's life-span close to its as yet undetermined biological limit.

There is reason to believe that a limit does exist. Even if one could erase the cumulative wear and tear that affects the aging organism, it seems probable that the cells themselves are not programmed for perpetual activity. The differences in the life-spans of various animals suggest some such natural limit. The changes that are observed in the tissues of animals that undergo metamorphosis—for example insects—are indicative of the programmed extinction of certain tissues. So is the failure of the human ovaries at menopause, long before other vital organs give out. Leonard Hayflick of the Stanford University School of Medicine has reported that the cells in cultures of human embryonic connective tissue will divide some 50 times and then die. If growth is interrupted by plunging the culture into liquid nitrogen, the cells will resume growth on thawing, continue through the remainder of their 50 divisions and then die. Although one may question whether the cells are not affected by adverse environmental influences, Hayflick's studies support the notion of programmed death. Only cancer cells seem capable of eternal life in culture. One familiar line of cancer cells, the "HeLa" strain, has often been the subject of cell-culture studies; it originated as a cervical cancer 21 years ago and has been maintained in culture ever since.

As investigations and speculations seek an answer to the question of the natural limits of life, other workers have noted that the giant molecules of living matter themselves age. Collagen, the main protein of connective tissue, constitutes approximately 30 percent of all the protein in the human body. With advancing age collagen molecules show a spontaneous increase in the cross-linking of their subunits, a process that increases their rigidity and reduces their solubility. Such a stiffening of this important structural component of our bodies might underlie such classic features of aging as rigidity of blood vessels, resistance to blood flow, reduced delivery of blood through hardened arteries and, as a final consequence, the loss of cells and of function. Other giant molecules, including the DNA molecule that stores the genetic information and the RNA molecule that reads out the stored message, may also be subject to spontaneous cross-linking that would eventually prevent the normal self-renewal of tissues.

A new area in aging research appears to be opening up in studies on the immune system of the body. In addition to providing antibodies against bacteria or foreign substances introduced into the body, the immune system recognizes and destroys abnormal or foreign cells. When these functions of the immune system diminish, as happens with advancing age, there may be errors in the system that result in antibodies that attack and destroy normal body cells or impair their function. The net result of this disturbed activity of the immune system, like the cross-linking of collagen, would be what is recognized as the aging process.

Takashi Makinodan of the Baltimore City Hospitals thinks that methods of rejuvenating the immune system are possible. The hope that some medicine will be discovered that can block the fundamental process of aging, however, seems to me very remote until the nature of the aging process is far better understood.

Much research is needed before such an understanding can be attained. It is nonetheless encouraging that aging research is finding increased interest and support in several countries. It is also encouraging to perceive a parallel interest in the aged among scientists, physicians, economists, politicians and others. To consider any extension of the human life-span without a serious effort to anticipate and plan for the impact of increased longevity on society would be entirely irresponsible.

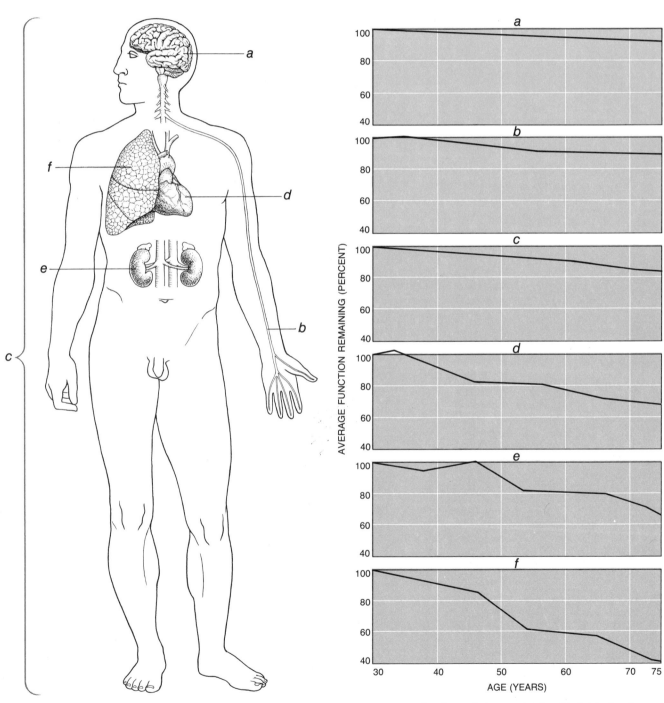

LOSS OF FUNCTION with increasing age does not occur at the same rate in all organs and systems. Graphs (right) show loss as a percentage, with the level of function at age 30 representing 100 percent. Thus brain weight (a) has diminished to 92 percent of its age-30 value by age 75 and nerve-conduction velocity (b) to about 90 percent. The basal metabolic rate (c) has diminished to 84 percent, cardiac output at rest (d) to 70 percent, filtration rate of the kidneys (e) to 69 percent and maximum breathing capacity (f) to 43 percent. Diseases, however, rather than gradual diminution of function, are at present the chief barrier to extended longevity.

IV

Dying

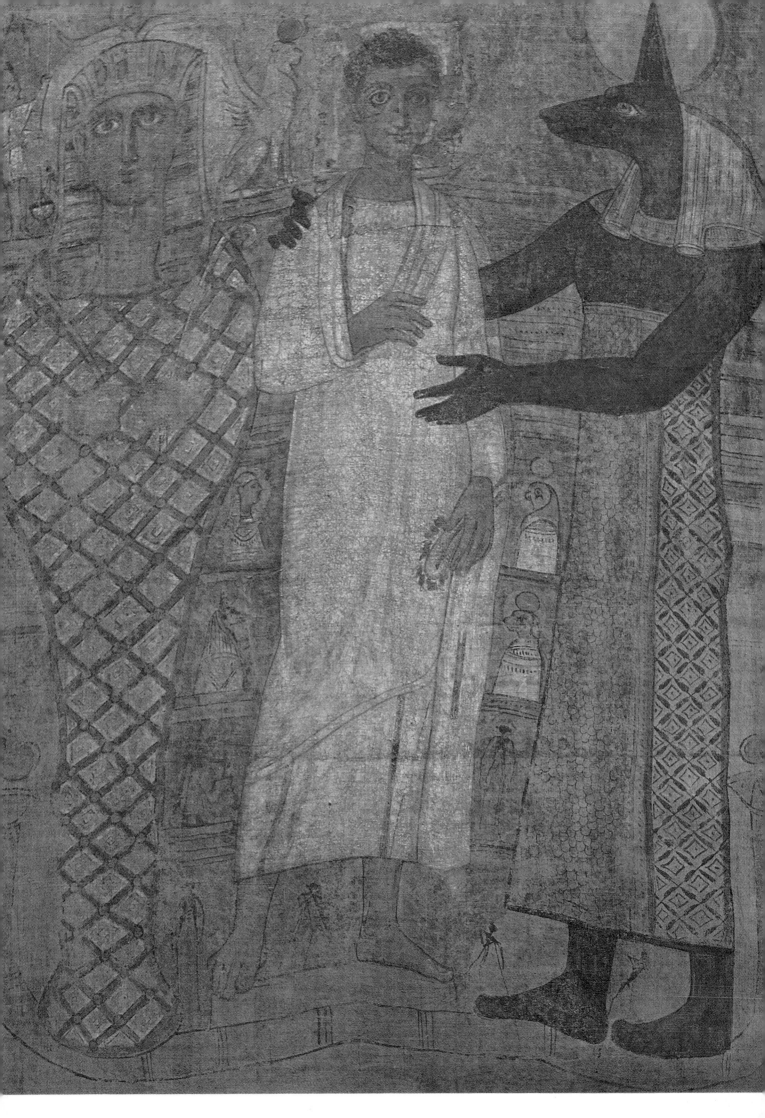

Dying

ROBERT S. MORISON

In the industrialized countries nearly two-thirds of the deaths are now associated with the infirmities of old age. Medicine can fend off death, but in doing so it often merely prolongs agony

The contemplation of death in the 20th century can tell us a good deal about what is right and what is wrong with modern medicine. At the beginning of the century death came to about 15 percent of all newborn babies in their first year and to perhaps another 15 percent before adolescence. Nowadays fewer than 2 percent die in their first year and the great majority will live to be over 70.

Most of the improvement can be explained by changes in the numbers of deaths from infectious disease, brought about in large part by a combination of better sanitation, routine immunization and specific treatment with chemotherapeutic drugs or antibiotics. Also important, although difficult to quantify, are improvements in the individual's nonspecific resistance that are attributable to improved nutrition and general hygiene.

Infectious diseases typically attack younger people. Equally typically, although not uniformly, they either cause death in a relatively short time or disappear completely, leaving the individual much as he was before. That is what makes death from infection particularly poignant. The large number of people who used to die of infection died untimely deaths; they had not lived long enough to enjoy the normal human experiences of love, marriage, supporting a family, painting a picture or discovering a scientific truth.

The medical profession and the individual physician clearly had every in-

centive to struggle endlessly against deaths of this kind. Every triumph over an untimely death was rewarded by the high probability of complete recovery and a long, happy and productive life. No wonder the profession developed an ethic that placed a preponderant emphasis on preserving life at all costs. No wonder also that it became preoccupied with the spectacular advances in science and technology that made such triumphs possible.

Nevertheless, it is still clear that we must all die sometime. As a matter of fact, the age at which the last member of a cohort, or age class, dies is now much the same as it was in biblical times. Whereas life expectancy at birth has improved by perhaps two and a half times, life expectancy at 70 has changed very little. (It is now approximately 12 years.) The difference is that in earlier times relatively few people managed to reach 70, whereas under present conditions nearly two-thirds of the population reach that age. As a result most people no longer die of some quick, acute illness but of the chronic deteriorations of old age. Only very recently has the general public or even the medical profession begun to realize that the attitudes and techniques developed in the battle against untimely death may not be entirely appropriate in helping the aged patient adapt to changed physiological and psychological circumstances.

The progress of technology puts in the physician's hands a constantly in-

creasing number of things he can do for and to his aging patients. In the jargon of modern policy, the "options" have been greatly increased and the problem of therapy has become largely a problem of choice. Modern students of decision theory point out that all methods of choice making reduce ultimately to the making of value judgments. When a pediatrician encounters an otherwise normal child with a life-threatening sore throat, the value judgment is simple and immediate. The life is obviously worth saving at all costs and the only choice to be made is what antibiotic to use. At the other end of life, however, most patients present a varied mosaic of diminished and disordered function. For a man or woman over a certain age there is no such thing as complete recovery. Treatment directed at supporting one vital system may simply bring into greater prominence a more awkward or more painful disorder. Furthermore, many of the treatment options, unlike the treatment of acute infections that may threaten premature death, are far from simple and inexpensive. Instead they are often cumbersome, painful and costly. The art, moreover, is constantly changing, so that it is hard to estimate the probable results of some of the most elaborate procedures.

For example, in managing the course of a patient with chronic cardiovascular disease the physician has available more or less conventional drugs that can strengthen and regularize the heartbeat, reduce the accumulation of excess fluid in the tissues, moderate the blood pressure and relieve the pain of reduced circulation to the heart muscle. These results can be achieved rather simply, and such treatment has for years prolonged and enhanced the quality of the life of many people over 60. Now, however, the physician must also weigh the proba-

DIVINE PERSONIFICATION OF DEATH, the jackal-headed Egyptian god Anubis grasps the tunic-clad soul of a young man in the painting of a funeral scene on the opposite page. The cloth-wound mummy bundle (*left*) contains the man's embalmed body. The exaggerated eyes of the central figure foreshadow the conventions of portrait painting during Egypt's Coptic and Byzantine period (A.D. 395–641) but the Roman tunic shows the painting belongs to the period of Roman rule (30 B.C.–A.D. 395). The painting is in the Louvre.

ble results of operations to install new heart valves, replace arteries or substitute pacemakers, all at a substantial risk to the patient's life and with the certainty of considerable pain and disability. At the end of this line is the transplantation of an entire heart, with so many risks and costs that its benefits currently tempt even the most courageous only rarely.

If the disease process leaves the heart relatively untouched and concentrates on the central nervous system, other possibilities assert themselves. Medical technology can now substitute for all the life-supporting functions of the nervous system. Tubes into either the gastrointestinal tract or a vein take the place of eating, a similar tube into the bladder takes the place of normal elimination and an artificial respirator takes the place of breathing. Various electronic devices can even keep the heart beating for weeks or months beyond its appointed time.

Thus it has come about that most therapeutic decisions for people above a certain age are not life-or-death decisions in any simple either-or sense. Inevitably the physician, the patient himself (if he is in a state to do so) or the patient's family must make more or less explicit judgments of the probable quality of the life that remains, as well as its probable length.

In this changed situation the severer critics of the medical profession go to considerable length to debunk the traditional mystery and wisdom of the physician as a decision maker. Among other things, they point out that there is nothing in the technological training of physicians that equips them to deal with questions of ethical, aesthetic or human value. Some even favor legislation removing life-or-death decisions entirely from the hands of the physician and giving them to an ombudsman or to a committee of moral philosophers.

Even the closest friends of medicine

must admit that the profession has brought much of the current criticism on itself by failing to maintain the balance between the technological and the humane that characterized the best physicians from the days of Hippocrates to roughly those of Sir William Osler (1849–1919). In a way physicians have been seduced, if not actually betrayed, by their very competence. They can do a great deal for their patients at a purely technological level and at the same time they face nothing but uncertainties when they confront the ineluctable ills of the spirit. Is it any wonder they rejoice in the one and neglect the other?

I have approached the problem of terminal illness, or the dying patient, in this somewhat circuitous fashion in order to show that the problems surrounding the deathbed are not quite so unprecedented or so unconnected with the rest of medicine as to require the development of entirely new attitudes or perhaps even a new profession of "thanatolo-

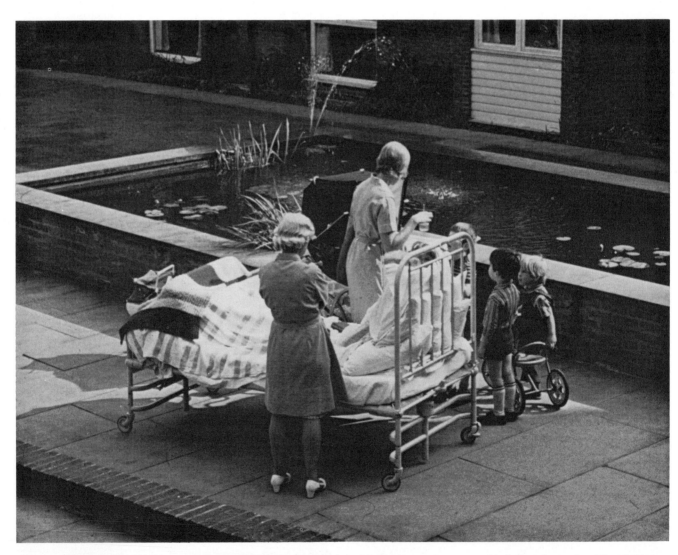

DEATH WITH DIGNITY is a primary objective at the English hospice St. Christopher's, site of the garden pool seen in this photograph. One of the terminally sick patients has been given a change of scene by moving his bed to the garden. The children at the bedside, pupils at a day-care center provided for dependents of the hospice staff, are welcomed by the patients as companions.

gists." Dying is continuous with living, and the questions that are now asked with such insistence at the bedside of the dying should also be at least in the back of the mind of those who attend the living in earlier stages. The physician must consider the quality of the life he is struggling to preserve and the probable effects of his therapy on this quality, whatever the age of the patient. He should also know how to help a patient of any age to accept circumstances that cannot be changed. The so-called terminally ill patient simply represents the limiting case. In this instance the value questions have become paramount.

For reasons that are not all easy to identify the past few years have seen an astonishing increase in public attention to death and dying. A recent bibliography listing the titles of both books and papers in scholarly journals on the subject is several pages long. It is a rare daily newspaper or popular periodical that has not published one such article or several. Approaches to the topic may be roughly separated into two classes: those that deal with making the patient's last days as physically and psychologically comfortable as possible and those that discuss the propriety of allowing or helping the patient to die at an appropriate time. Let us turn first to the care of the terminally ill.

Students of the process of dying have long emphasized the loneliness of the dying person. Not only is he destined to go where no one wants to follow but also the people around him prefer to pretend that the journey is really not going to take place. The practice of placing familiar articles and even animals, servants and wives in the tomb or on the funeral pyre of the departed is testimony to man's desire to assuage the loneliness beyond. In "The Death of Ivan Ilych" Leo Tolstoy has given the classic description of the conspiracy of denial that so often surrounds the dying. The situation has certainly been made worse by the technological changes since Tolstoy's day. Then, at least, most people died at home, many of them surrounded by family and friends. Even if these attendants were primarily concerned with what would happen to themselves, as were those awaiting the death of the old Count Bezhukoi that Tolstoy also portrayed, they not only kept the patient from being physically alone but also made him quite conscious of being the center of attention.

Nowadays only a minority of people die at home, and the number is decreasing. Precise figures are hard to obtain,

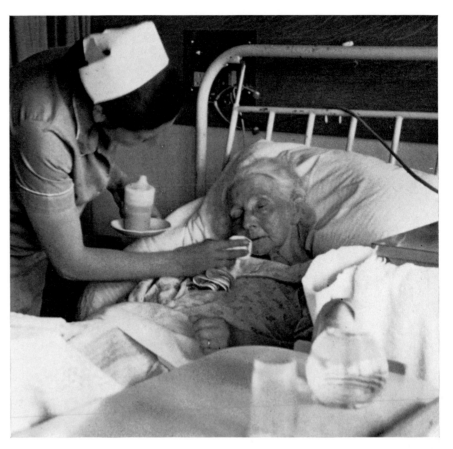

ELDERLY PATIENT at St. Christopher's is attended by one of the nursing staff. The age of the patient is greater than is usual among the dying who comprise the clientele of the hospice. The patients range in age from 16 to the 90's but most are between 55 and 65.

but the scattered studies that have been made agree that about half of all deaths occur in large general hospitals and a smaller but increasing number in nursing homes. Probably fewer than a third die at home, at work or in public places.

The past few years have seen a growing awareness that the big general hospital is not a very good place to die. Even though such hospitals have large staffs, most of these professionals are preoccupied with administrative matters and with the increasingly complicated technical aspects of keeping people alive. Surrounded by these busybodies, the dying patient is more often than not psychologically isolated. Recognizing that such an atmosphere is bad both for patients and for younger physicians in training, a few inspired physicians have developed special programs to instruct members of the hospital staff in the needs of the dying patient. Such efforts have been received with enthusiasm by the still quite limited numbers of physicians and students who have been exposed to them.

The usefulness of training hospital staff members to deal with the dying patient is a concept that is now spreading throughout the country. There is substantial hope that the next generation of

physicians, nurses and administrators will be much more understanding and helpful in meeting the special needs of the dying than their predecessors were. One of the leaders in this movement is an Illinois psychiatrist, Elisabeth K. Ross. In an effort to inject something approaching methodological rigor into her understanding and teaching of the needs of the dying, she has distinguished five stages exhibited by dying patients: denial, anger, bargaining (usually with God), depression and acceptance. This effort toward intellectualization of the problem is admirable; at the same time it is probably true that what has been most influential in alleviating the loneliness of the dying is the warmth of Dr. Ross's sympathy and the intensity of her dedication to the effort.

A high proportion of the patients in nursing homes are destined to die there or to be removed only at the very last minute for intensive hospital care, yet few of these institutions appear to have given much thought to the special problems of the dying. The most striking exceptions are provided by what in England are called "hospices." The best-known of them is St. Christopher's, outside London. It was started by a physician who was also trained as a nurse. She appears to have combined the best of both professions in developing arrangements for taking care of seriously ill patients and providing a warm and understanding atmosphere for them. Because many of the patients at St. Christopher's suffer from malignant disease, special emphasis is put on the alleviation of pain. It has been found that success depends not only on providing the right drugs at the right time but also on developing an attitude of understanding, confidence and hope. Psychological support involves, among other things, deinstitutionalizing the atmosphere by encouraging members of the family, including children and grandchildren, both to "visit the patient" in a formal sense and to carry on such activities as may be usual for their age, so that the patient feels surrounded by ongoing normal life. Everyone who has observed the program or has been privileged to participate in it speaks appreciatively and even enthusiastically about its achievements.

Hospices also serve as centers for an active home-care program that is demonstrating the practicality of tending to many dying patients in the home, provided that the physical arrangements are satisfactory and that specialized help from outside is available for a few hours a day. Unfortunately most insurance plans, including the otherwise enlightened National Health Service in Britain, have tended to emphasize hospital care to the detriment of adequate support for proper care in the home.

Recent studies of home care for seriously ill patients suggest that in many cases it can be not only more satisfactory emotionally than hospital care but also considerably less costly. Much more information is needed before administrators of health plans can determine precisely how many and what kinds of personnel should be available for how long to deal with various kinds of home situation. Similarly, a few preliminary surveys of the technological ways of adapting the American home for the care of the chronically ill have been made. Here again there is enough information to suggest the importance of funds for special types of beds and wheelchairs, the installation of plumbing within easy range of the sickbed and so on. The data, however, are not yet precise enough to allow adequate planning or the calculation of insurance premiums adequate to cover such services.

In spite of the potential emotional and economic benefits of home care one cannot overlook the fact that many social and technological changes have made illness and death at home very different from what they were in the days of Ivan Ilych and Count Bezhukoi. It is not appropriate here to try to cast up an account of the costs and benefits of such factors as rising social and geographic mobility and the transition from the extended family to the nuclear family. When these costs are counted, however, it may be well to include mention of the increasing difficulty in finding a good place to grow old and die.

Let us next examine the question of when it becomes appropriate to die. No matter how considerate the physician, how supportive the institutional atmosphere, how affectionately concerned the family and friends or how well-adjusted the patient himself, there comes a time when all those involved must ask themselves just how much sense it makes to continue vigorously trying to postpone the inevitable. Regrettably the literature addressed to the topics of death and dying often seems preoccupied more with dissecting the various ethical and legal niceties surrounding the moment and manner of death than with what one can do to make the last few months or years of life as rewarding as possible. No doubt this preoccupation is prompted by an apparent conflict between ancient taboos on the one hand and certain obvious commonsense considerations on the other.

Now, virtually no one who has thought about the matter at all, from John Doe to the Pope, feels that any absolute moral or legal obligation requires one to do everything one knows how to do in order to preserve the life of a severely deteriorated patient beyond hope of recovery. Indeed, in actual practice it now seems probable that only a small minority of patients have everything possible done for them right up to the moment of death. The difficulties, then, are not with the general principle but with how to arrange the details. First and foremost in presenting themselves are the theoretical and even metaphysical problems involved in the ways that men of goodwill attempt to justify ac-

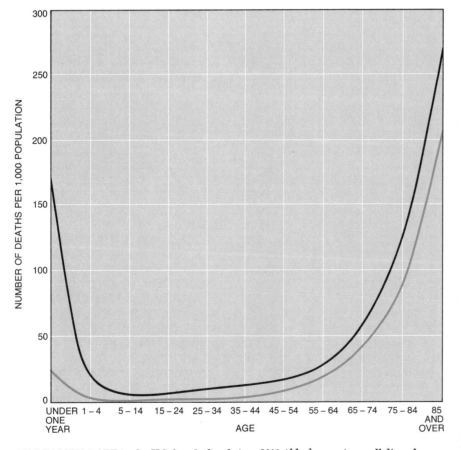

MORTALITY RATE in the U.S. has declined since 1900 (*black curve*), paralleling changes in the age composition of the population. The 1900 rate was 17.2 per 1,000. By 1954 it had dropped to 9.2, a record low, and in 1966 (*colored curve*) it stood at 9.5. As the curves show, the outstanding differences between 1900 and 1966 lie in the greatly reduced number of deaths during the first year of life and, to a lesser extent, during the years after the age of 55.

tions that appear to violate the taboo against killing. Second, there are practical questions to be answered. How can the individual make sure that his wishes are carried out? Who is to make the decision if the patient is no longer competent to do so? What are the physician's responsibilities? What, for that matter, are his possible liabilities? How far should society go in attempting to protect the rights and regulate the behavior of the various parties?

No more than an outline of the theoretical problems can be presented here. Current discussion centers principally on three issues. First is the definition of death. Next is the difference, if any, between negative and positive euthanasia and last is the definition of "extraordinary means."

The possibility of redefining death came into prominence a few years ago when a group of Boston physicians grew concerned about precisely when it was appropriate to remove a prospective donor's organs for transplantation. It rapidly became clear that "defining" death, for whatever purpose, is a complicated philosophical matter that admits of no easy resolution. What the members of the Boston group actually did was to devise an operational redefinition of the criteria to be applied in declaring that a person has died. The major difficulty they faced arose from the purely technical fact that it is now possible to maintain the function of the heart and the lungs by artificial means. The failure of these two vital functions can therefore no longer be regarded in all cases as the paramount criteria for pronouncing death, as was once set forth in all conventional medical-legal texts.

The Boston group instead recommended the use of a set of signs testifying to an essentially complete failure of a third set of functions: those of the nervous system. This proposal has been received with approval by a large number of physicians, theologians and lawyers, and has now been included in the law of several states. The criteria as they stand are extremely rigid and involve the death of essentially all levels of the nervous system. They thus seem entirely adequate both to protect the patient against premature assaults in order to retrieve viable organs and at the same time to guard him against unduly zealous attempts to maintain elementary vital signs in the name of therapy.

There is another class of patients, however, in whom elementary vital signs have not failed, although the higher brain functions—thinking, communicat-

TO MY FAMILY, MY PHYSICIAN, MY CLERGYMAN, MY LAWYER —

If the time comes when I can no longer take part in decisions for my own future, let this statement stand as the testament of my wishes:

If there is no reasonable expectation of my recovery from physical or mental disability,

I, _____

request that I be allowed to die and not be kept alive by artificial means or heroic measures. Death is as much a reality as birth, growth, maturity and old age—it is the one certainty. I do not fear death as much as I fear the indignity of deterioration, dependence and hopeless pain. I ask that medication be mercifully administered to me for terminal suffering even if it hastens the moment of death.

This request is made after careful consideration. Although this document is not legally binding, you who care for me will, I hope, feel morally bound to follow its mandate. I recognize that it places a heavy burden of responsibility upon you, and it is with the intention of sharing that responsibility and of mitigating any feelings of guilt that this statement is made.

Signed _____

Date _____

Witnessed by:

_____

"LIVING WILL" is a formal request prepared by the Euthanasia Educational Council. It informs the signer's family or others who may be concerned of the signer's wish to avoid the use of "heroic measures" to maintain life in the event of irreversible illness.

ing with others and even consciousness itself—have departed. Such a patient constitutes a most distressing problem to families and physicians, and it has been suggested that a further revision of the criteria for a pronouncement of death might be used to justify the termination of active treatment in such cases. The idea is that what is really human and important about the individual resides in the upper levels of the nervous system, and that these attributes indeed die with the death of the forebrain.

The presumed merit of such a revision grows out of the way it avoids the basic ethical problem; obviously it makes no sense to go on treating what can rationally be defined as a corpse. The weight of opinion, however, seems to be against dealing with the question of cerebral incapacity in this oblique way. From several standpoints it seems preferable to face up to the fact that under these circumstances a patient may still be living in some sense, but that the obligation to treat the living is neither absolute nor inexorable.

No less a moral authority than the Pope appears to have lent his weight to this view and even to have spoken for most Christians when he announced a few years ago that the physician is not required to use "extraordinary means" to maintain the spark of life in a deteriorated patient with no evident possibility of recovery. Nevertheless, serious ambiguities still remain. At first the Vatican's phraseology appears to have been designed to allow the withdrawal of "heroic" and relatively novel procedures such as defibrillation, cardiac massage and artificial respiration. More subtle analysts point out that there is no absolute scale of extraordinariness, and that what is or is not extraordinary can only be judged in relation to the condition of a given individual. Hence there is nothing extraordinary about using all possible means to keep alive a young mother who has suffered multiple fractures, severe hemorrhages and temporary unconsciousness. Conversely, the term extraordinary may well be applied to relatively routine procedures such as intravenous feeding if the patient is elderly, has deteriorated and has little hope of improvement. Thus the most active proponents of the doctrine of extraordinary means clearly interpret "extraordinary" to mean "inappropriate in the circumstances." Although many people who hold this position would disagree, it is not easy for an outsider to distinguish their interpretation from advocacy of what is sometimes called "negative euthanasia."

Negative euthanasia refers to withdrawal of treatment from a patient who as a result is likely to die somewhat earlier than he otherwise would. Many thoughtful and sensitive people who favor the principle dislike the term because it suggests that treatment is being withdrawn with an actual, if unspoken, intent to shorten the patient's life. These critics, who place a high value on the taboo against taking life, prefer to regard the withdrawal of active therapy as simply a matter of changing from a therapeutic regime that is inappropriate to one that is more appropriate under the circumstances. If death then supervenes, it is not regarded as the result of anything the physician has or has not done but simply as a consequence of the underlying illness. Thus the physician and those who have perhaps participated in his decision are protected from the fear that they are "playing God" or from similar feelings of guilt.

Many of those who favor negative euthanasia also recognize that appropriate care of the terminally ill may include "positive" procedures, such as giving morphine (which, among other effects, may advance the moment of death). Invoking what is known in Catholic circles as the doctrine, or law, of double effect, they regard such positive actions as permissible as long as the conscious intent is to achieve some licit purpose such as the relief of pain. This view in turn requires the drawing of an important moral distinction between "awareness of probable result" and "intent."

Other moralists, such as the blunter and more forthright proponents of what is called situational ethics, may dismiss such subtleties as irrelevant logic-chopping. In their view it is a mistake to extend the generalized taboos and abstract principles of the past to encompass the peculiarities of the 20th-century death scene. They prefer to focus attention on the scene itself and to do what seems best in terms of the probable results for all concerned. Perhaps not surprisingly, the situational ethicist, who derives much of his philosophical base from classical utilitarian, or consequential, ethics, sees relatively little difference between negative and positive euthanasia, that is, between allowing to die and causing to die.

For the sake of completeness let me inject my own opinion that although there may be only a trivial intellectual distinction between negative and positive euthanasia, it seems unwise and in any event useless at this time to enter into an elaborate defense of positive euthanasia. Although the principle has its enthusiastic advocates, their number is strictly limited. The overwhelming majority of physicians and certainly a substantial majority of laymen instinctively recoil from such active measures as prescribing a known poison or injecting a large bubble into a vein. There seems to be a point where simple human reactions supersede both legal sanction and rational analysis. As an example, very few New York physicians or nurses are anxious to exercise the right given them by the laws of the state to perform abortions as late as the 24th week of pregnancy. Furthermore, it appears that as a practical matter negative euthanasia, or the withdrawal of all active therapy except the provision of narcotics to subdue restlessness and pain, will in any case be followed in a reasonable length of time by the coming of what Osler termed near the turn of the century the "old man's friend": a peaceful death from bronchial pneumonia. Thus, in the terminology of the law courts, we need not reach the most difficult question.

In view of the prevailing theoretical uncertainties, it is not surprising that what is done to or for the dying patient varies widely from place to place and from physician to physician. It is impossible to be precise because very few scientific observations have been made. Perhaps the most careful study is one conducted by Diana Crane of the University of Pennsylvania, who asked a large number of physicians and surgeons what they would probably do in a series of precisely outlined clinical situations. From this and more anecdotal evidence it seems clear that very few do everything possible to prolong the lives of all their patients. At the other extreme, even fewer physicians would appear to employ active measures with the avowed intent of shortening life. In between there is an enormous range of decisions: to give or not to give a transfusion, to prescribe an antibiotic or a sulfa drug, to attach or disconnect a respirator or an artificial kidney, to install a cardiac pacemaker or to let the battery of one that is already installed run down. The overall impression gained both by the informed observer and by the sometimes despairing layman is that the median of all these activities lies rather far toward officiously keeping alive.

The reasons are obvious enough: the momentum of a professional tradition of preserving life at all costs, the reluctance of the physician and the layman to ignore ancient taboos or to impair the value of such positive concepts as the sanctity of life, and the ambiguities of the love-hate relationship between parents and children or husbands and wives. Finally, there is the continuing uncertainty about the legal position of a physician who might be charged with hastening the death of a patient by acts of either omission or commission.

Up to now, at least, the legal deterrent appears to have been something of a chimera. A conscientious search of the available literature in English has un-

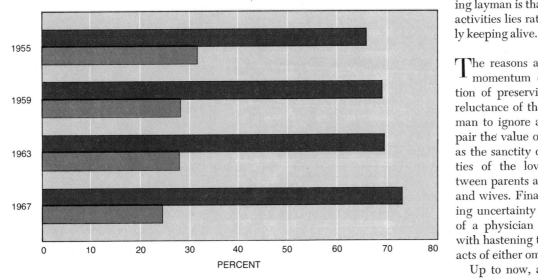

1955
1959
1963
1967

0   10   20   30   40   50   60   70   80
PERCENT

FEWER DEATHS AT HOME (*color*) than in institutions (*gray*) has been the trend in New York City since 1955. That year more than 31 percent of deaths occurred at home (the national average was about 40 percent), but by 1967 home deaths had fallen below 25 percent.

covered not one criminal action charging that a physician omitted treatment with the intent to shorten life. Indeed, there are surprisingly few actions that charge positive euthanasia. Even in the few actions that have been lodged, juries have shown a reluctance to convict when there is evidence that the action was undertaken in good faith to put the patient on the far side of suffering.

Approaching the problem from a somewhat different angle, although the definitive examples are few, there appears to be general agreement that the adult patient in full possession of his senses has every right to refuse treatment. It is somewhat less certain that such refusal is binding after a patient loses legal competence. Even less clear is the status of the expressed wish of a potential patient with respect to what he would want done in certain hypothetical future circumstances. Efforts to clarify the status of such communications, sometimes called "living wills," with physicians and relatives are being actively pursued.

Important though it may be to establish the rights and privileges of those foresighted enough to want to participate in the design of their own death, it must be admitted that such individuals now constitute only a trivial part of the population. The great majority prefer not to think about their own death in any way. Indeed, most people do not even leave a will directing what to do with their material possessions.

What, then, can be done for that large number of people likely to slip into an unanticipated position of indignity on a deathbed surrounded by busybodies with tubes and needles in their hands, ready to substitute a chemical or mechanical device for every item in the human inventory except those that make human life significant? In such instances, under ideal, or perhaps I should say idyllic, circumstances the attending physician would have known the patient and his family for a long time. Further, he would have sensed their conscious and unconscious wishes and needs, and drawing on his accumulated skills and wisdom, he would conduct the last illness so as to maximize the welfare of all concerned. Unfortunately under modern conditions few families have a regular physician of any kind and even fewer physicians possess the hypothetical virtues I have outlined.

However that may be, at least three approaches to the problem are being actively pursued at present. Foremost among them is the active discussion I have referred to. Not only the professional journals but also the monthly, weekly and daily press are publishing numerous articles on death and dying. Radio and television programs have followed suit, and it must be a rare church discussion group that has not held at least one meeting devoted to death with dignity. At the very least such discussion must remove some of the reluctance to speak of death or even think about it. At best it must improve the possibility of communication and understanding between the patient and the physician. The resulting change in the climate of opinion cannot fail to make it easier to discard outmoded taboos in favor of the common sense of contemporary men.

Second, and equally important, are the formal and informal efforts to improve the education of physicians by redressing the imbalance between technical skill and human wisdom that has grown up during the present century. In addition to the kind of clinical concern for the dying exemplified by Dr. Ross, many medical schools are converting their courses in medical ethics from a guild-oriented preoccupation with fee splitting and other offenses against the in-group to a genuine concern for ethical values in the treatment of patients.

Third, there are the more formal attempts to clarify rights, responsibilities and roles by means of legislation. Part of this effort is directed at establishing the obligation of a physician to follow the expressed wishes of his patient or, at the very least, at protecting the physician from liability if he does so. Other legislative proposals stem from a more or less explicit conviction that death is too important a matter to be left to physicians. Difficulty is often encountered, however, in finding a satisfactory alternative, and there is now much discussion of the relative merits of assigning ultimate authority to the next-of-kin, to an ombudsman or to a committee of social scientists, philosophers and theologians.

It is too early to predict how such suggestions will turn out, but there are some reasons for feeling that it may be well to go slow in formalizing what is bound to be a difficult situation and instead to redouble efforts toward developing the capacity of medical men and laymen to deal informally with the problem. In actual practice the conduct of a drawn-out terminal illness involves a series of small decisions, based on repeated evaluations of the physical and emotional condition of the patient and the attitudes, hopes and fears of his family and friends. It is not easy to see how an outsider such as an ombudsman, much less a committee, can be very easily fitted into what is typically an unobtrusive incremental process. Concrete evidence on this point may be found with respect to the beginning of life in the attempts by opponents of contraception to inject either a sheriff or a bureaucrat, so to speak, into the bedroom. These attempts have not proved satisfactory and are more and more being denounced by the courts as invasions of privacy.

As long as progress is being made at the informal, grass-roots level, it may be just as well to refrain from drafting tidy legislative solutions to problems so profound. Whatever else may be said, it is obvious that changing attitudes toward death and dying provide an excellent paradigm of how changing technologies force on us the consideration of equally significant changes in value systems and social institutions.

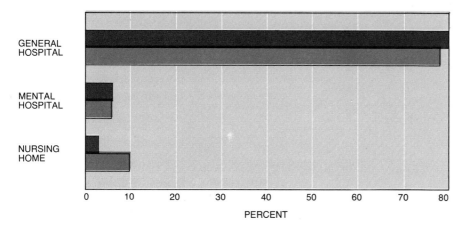

DEATHS AWAY FROM HOME in the U.S. during two recent years, 1949 (*gray*) and 1958 (*color*), followed quite similar patterns. The large majority of deaths occurred in general hospitals and a small number occurred in mental hospitals. A possible trend toward increased use of self-styled "nursing homes" as depots for the irreversibly sick is seen in the rise in the number of deaths in such institutions from 1949 to 1958. These data and those in the preceding graphs were furnished by Monroe Lerner of Johns Hopkins University.

V

The Ills of Man

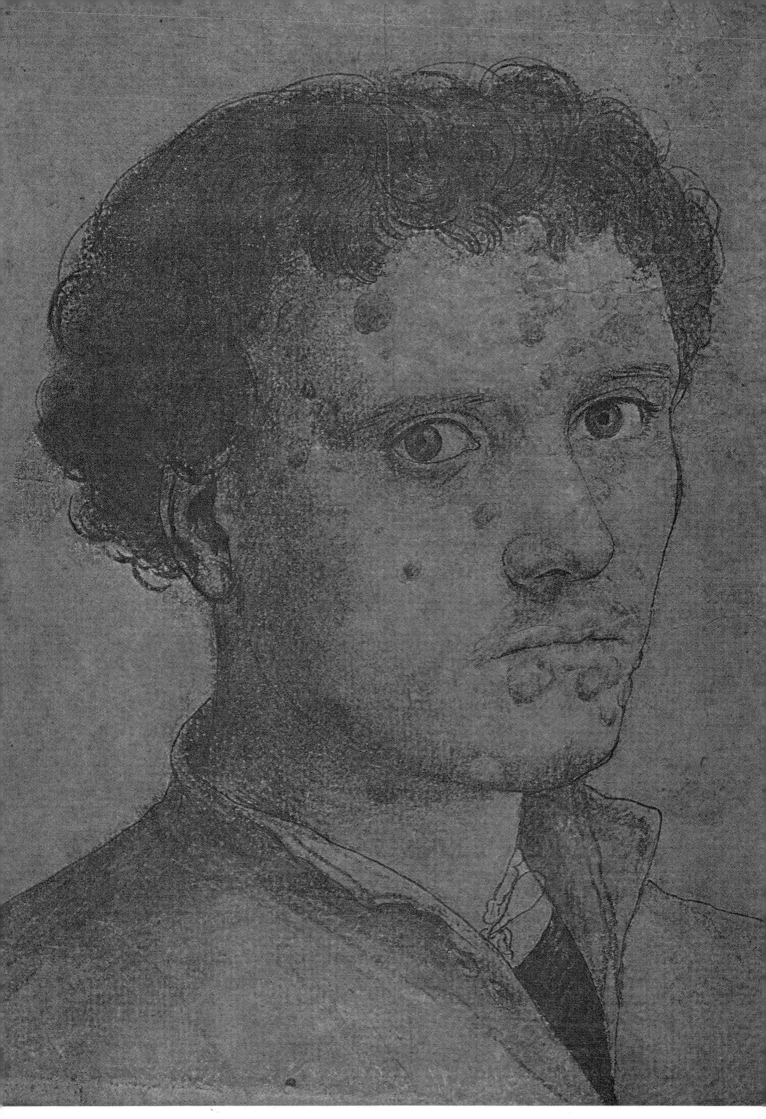

The Ills of Man

JOHN H. DINGLE

The most prevalent diseases are not the well-known causes of death. Precisely what they are depends to a surprising degree on whether they are perceived by patients, by physicians or by vital statisticians

To the average "well informed" reader in the U.S. today cancer, heart attacks and acts of violence, including accidents and homicides, must seem to be the preponderant ills of modern man. To be sure, these few afflictions are among the leading causes of death, the terminal event in the lives of all people. They nonetheless represent only a small proportion of man's ills, which are legion and diverse in nature, varying, for example, with race, ethnic background, geographic location, time, causation, severity and outcome. Some are inherent in man's genetic makeup; others are the inevitable results of conflicts with his environment; still others are man-made. Some ills, although seemingly minor or even trivial at first, can lead through recurrence or progression to serious states of chronic disease and to death. Many ills are perceived only by the person himself, as a sense of "not feeling well"; they cannot be objectively determined by the physician even with his modern diagnostic tools, nor can they be labeled as "diseases" with classical physiological, metabolic, structural or pathologic symptoms. Other ills, of course, can be diagnosed as well-known and well-described diseases or syndromes, or as new or newly recognized disease states.

Clearly the ills of man could be described and discussed from so many points of view that volumes, not mere pages, would be required. I propose, therefore, to limit the subject to four somewhat arbitrary general headings and under each heading to give examples, where they are appropriate, of the dynamic nature of illness as shown by its natural history and by the effect of deliberate intervention by man. The general headings I have chosen are (1) the ills of man as perceived by people, (2) the ills of man as perceived by physicians, (3) the ills of man as perceived by people and physicians, and (4) the ills of man as perceived by compilers of vital statistics.

A community's knowledge of the health status of its people is vitally important, since healthy people are the community's fundamental resource and keeping people healthy, or restoring them to health, is one of its greatest problems. The most reliable data obtainable are needed not only to estimate the requirements both now and in the future for medical services and hospital beds but also to evaluate the human resources, the economic potentials and many other components of a complex society.

The development of health statistics has been and still is an extremely slow process, and for a good reason: the problem of measurement. To call many of the studies and surveys that have been done "health surveys" is in a sense a misnomer, since they are really "sickness surveys" derived typically from physicians' reports of communicable diseases (as required by many state laws) and from reports by hospitals, clinics, insurance companies and group medical plans. In addition there have been a few large illness surveys such as those carried out in the U.S. from 1935 to 1936, in Britain from 1944 to 1952 and in Canada from 1950 to 1951.

The real problem is to define "health" and its attributes. Alan Gregg of the Rockefeller Foundation emphasized the difficulty when he said that if you give almost any literate person a sheet of paper and ask him to list all the symptoms of disease he can think of in five minutes, he will write down at least a dozen, whereas if you ask him to list the symptoms of health, he can seldom name even one or two. The constitution of the World Health Organization defines health as "a state of complete physical, mental and social well-being and not merely the absence of disease and infirmity." That is an elegant statement, but unfortunately those who drafted it did not define their terms nor did they indicate how the terms could be made quantitative. So far no one else has, either, at least in any satisfactory way.

The Canadian Sickness Survey of 1950–1951 covered the 14 million Canadians alive during the survey year. On an average day about 85 percent of the population reported no sickness, not even minor ailments. Over the period of a year, however, the figure was reduced to 19.6 percent. Over a longer period the figure would undoubtedly be reduced to zero. Clearly new concepts and more data concerning "health" are needed.

The nationwide health survey carried out in the U.S. in 1935–1936 was an at-

HEAD OF A YOUNG MAN with an unspecified skin condition was drawn in the 16th century by Hans Holbein the Younger. The drawing, which is in the Fogg Art Museum at Harvard University, exemplifies one of the most common difficulties confronted by medical statisticians in seeking to catalogue the ills that flesh is heir to: the problem of classification. According to the Fogg Art Museum's publication *Works of Art from the Collection of Paul J. Sachs*, "for many years the drawing was called *Portrait of a Leper*. Leprosy was long a generic term for skin diseases. More than one distinguished dermatologist in recent years has diagnosed the young man's ailment as a case of *impetigo contagioso*." The drawing, which measures eight inches high by six inches wide, is rendered in chalk with pen outlines.

tempt to obtain comprehensive illness statistics for the general population. It was a prodigious effort, including interviews in 737,000 urban households, with the emphasis on disabling illnesses and chronic diseases. Although the data were reliable for a variety of purposes, the survey had the defect that it did not include rural and suburban populations. With the large-scale shifts in population accompanying World War II the statistics became obsolete.

In 1948 the U.S. Committee on Vital and Health Statistics was established, composed of the most highly qualified experts in the field in the country. That committee and its subcommittees stud-

ied and discussed the "problems in morbidity statistics, including chronic diseases and medical-care statistics, in order that morbidity data may be directly related to demographic factors." The recommendations of these committees led to the passage by Congress of the National Health Survey Act in 1956. That law authorized the Surgeon General of the Public Health Service to make continuing surveys and special studies of the population of the U.S. in order to determine the extent of illness and disability and related information, including the economic impact of such conditions. It also authorized and directed cooperation and consultation with

other interested Federal departments (such as the Department of Commerce and the Department of Labor), with state agencies and with various other public or private agencies, groups and individuals.

The primary component of the health survey is the household interview, which provides data based on a general sample of the population of the 50 states. The data thus originate with the people themselves, the only individuals involved who have all the needed facts: the fact of illness, the action taken as a result of the illness, the duration of the illness and the demographic and personal details. Special studies that have more direct objectives, such as a survey for a specific disease or in a local area, can be related to the basic information from the household interviews.

The interviewing process is continuous, the questions asked are changed or supplemented from time to time to obtain pertinent contemporary information, and the sample of households is changed at appropriate intervals so that no household is interviewed twice except for purposes of checking reliability. The Public Health Service determines the substantive content of the questionnaires, evaluates and interprets the data obtained and publishes the results in a series of reports titled Vital and Health Statistics. The Bureau of the Census participates in planning, selects the sample by a highly stratified, multistage probability design and collects and tabulates the data. The interviewers are specifically trained, as are their supervisors.

The questionnaires are all reviewed in Washington for errors and are then coded. Medical coding is one obvious difficulty, since many "illnesses" can be described only symptomatically and not diagnostically. To eliminate trivial episodes an illness is accepted as such only if medical attention was sought or if activity was restricted for one day or more. Medical coding for such conditions is initially done independently by two coders; differences, if any, are umpired by a coding expert. The *Manual of the International Statistical Classification of Diseases, Injuries, and Causes of Death* is used for classification. In general, almost all illnesses can be classified, at least under the broader classifications.

Let us now examine some selected data for 1970, based on a sample composed of approximately 37,000 households consisting of about 116,000 persons living at the time of the interview [*see illustration at left*]. The number of new acute conditions was 203.4 per 100

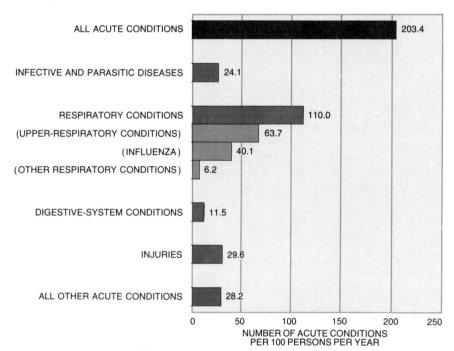

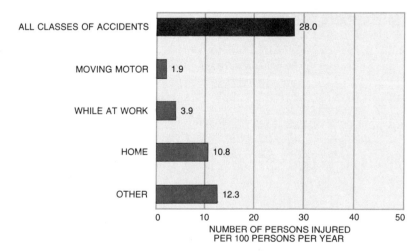

HEALTH-SURVEY FINDINGS provide a picture of the incidence of disease and accidents in the U.S. as perceived by the people themselves. The data summarized in these bar charts, published last year by the National Center for Health Statistics, are derived from a general survey conducted in 1970 of the population of the 50 states. The survey sample was composed of approximately 37,000 households consisting of about 116,000 people. The total number of new acute conditions for the year was 203.4 per 100 people, or slightly more than two per person. Accidents of various types accounted for about an eighth of the total.

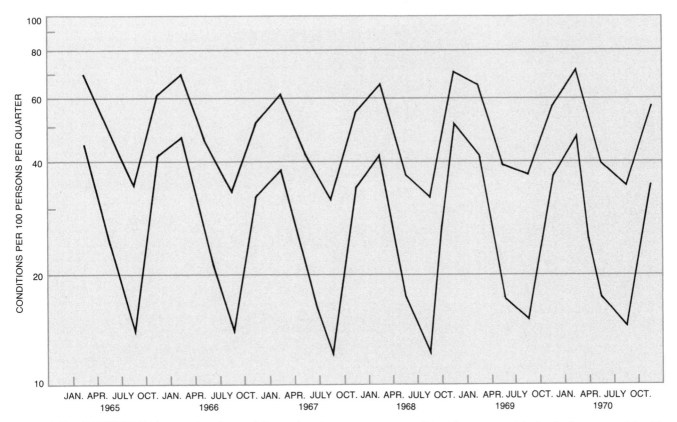

CONDITIONS PER 100 PERSONS PER QUARTER

JAN. APR. JULY OCT. JAN. APR. JULY OCT. JAN. APR. JULY OCT. JAN. APR. JULY OCT. JAN. APR. JULY OCT. JAN. APR. JULY OCT.
1965   1966   1967   1968   1969   1970

DOMINANT INFLUENCE of seasonal and annual fluctuations in the incidence of acute respiratory conditions (*lower curve*) in determining the shape of the curve representing the incidence of all new acute conditions (*upper curve*) is clearly demonstrated by this graph. The major contributors to this largest single disease category recorded in the U.S. survey are the common cold and influenza.

people for the year, or slightly more than two per person. By far the largest component was respiratory conditions, to which the common cold and influenza are the major contributors. This has been true each year since the survey began, and in fact the incidence of respiratory conditions determines the shape of the seasonal and annual curves for all conditions [*see illustration above*]. The subcategory "Other respiratory conditions" consists chiefly of pneumonia and bronchitis. "Infective and parasitic diseases" includes the common communicable diseases of childhood, worm infestations and miscellaneous viral infections. The remaining categories are self-explanatory.

The number of people suffering accidents was large, accounting for about an eighth of the total. Moving motor-vehicle accidents, however, were the smallest subcategory, involving slightly fewer than two per 100 people during the year, whereas house accidents occurred five times more frequently.

Days of disability from all causes remained essentially stable during the three years from the beginning of 1968 through the end of 1970. Limitation of all activity due to chronic conditions showed an increase of almost 1 percent in the total population between 1968 and 1970, and probably reflects the in-

crease in the number of people suffering from chronic diseases in an aging population.

These data are only a small fraction of those that can be found in the more than 200 reports from the National Center for Health Statistics based on information obtained from the National Health Survey and special studies and surveys.

Most physicians gain only a narrow and limited view of man's ailments from their experience in the practice of medicine. This statement is perhaps most obviously true for those who limit their practice to one or another of the specialties. Their patients are to a considerable extent referred to them by other physicians, although some undoubtedly select a specialist because of the belief that their problem and complaints lie within the realm of his specialty. The latter type of selection has become increasingly prevalent in this country because of the decline in the number of general practitioners, or family doctors, to whom the patient could go with his early complaints and who would guide the patient to an appropriate specialist, if necessary.

There are other factors that restrict the clinical experience of physicians. Among them are geographic location, ancillary medical facilities and time.

Time may often be the most important factor because there is a physical limit to the number of patients a physician can see and care for in a day, a week, a year or a lifetime. Thus a truly comprehensive view of man's ills as perceived by physicians must await the further collection and analysis of data from the physicians themselves. Such studies have been and are being made, but they are far from complete.

The type of physician whose experience in practice might come the closest to giving us a physician's picture of man's ailments, although it will be based on an extremely small group of people, is the general practitioner. Accordingly I have chosen to discuss briefly here some of the observations made by a British physician, John Fry, and published in his book *Profiles of Disease: A Study in the Natural History of Common Diseases*. Fry has been in general practice in a suburb of London for more than 20 years. He reports his experience in some detail from the period of 1947, when his practice population was some 3,000, to 1964, when it was 7,500. The median population, on which his calculations are generally based, was taken as the population at the mid-period of 1955.

In this population of almost 5,500 there was only a slight excess of females over males from the age of 20 years on.

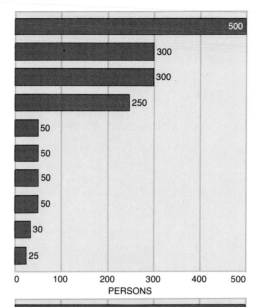

MINOR ILLNESS
UPPER-RESPIRATORY INFECTIONS — 500
COMMON DIGESTIVE DISORDERS — 300
SKIN DISORDERS — 300
MINOR EMOTIONAL DISORDERS — 250
ACUTE OTITIS MEDIA — 50
WAX IN EARS — 50
"ACUTE BACK" — 50
ACUTE URINARY INFECTIONS — 50
MIGRAINE — 30
HAY FEVER — 25

PERSONS (0, 100, 200, 300, 400, 500)

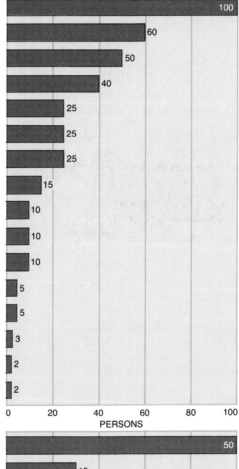

CHRONIC ILLNESS
CHRONIC RHEUMATISM (ALL FORMS) — 100
CHRONIC EMOTIONAL ILLNESS — 60
CHRONIC BRONCHITIS — 50
ANEMIA — 40
HYPERTENSION — 25
ASTHMA — 25
PEPTIC ULCER — 25
STROKES — 15
RHEUMATOID ARTHRITIS — 10
EPILEPSY — 10
DIABETES MELLITUS — 10
PULMONARY TUBERCULOSIS (OLD AND NEW) — 5
PERNICIOUS ANEMIA — 5
PARKINSONISM — 3
MULTIPLE SCLEROSIS — 2
MENTAL DEFICIENCY — 2

PERSONS (0, 20, 40, 60, 80, 100)

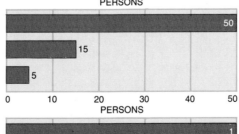

MAJOR ILLNESS
PNEUMONIA AND ACUTE BRONCHITIS — 50
CORONARY HEART DISEASES (NEW CASES 7) — 15
ACUTE APPENDICITIS — 5

PERSONS (0, 10, 20, 30, 40, 50)

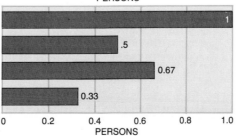

ALL NEW CANCERS
CANCER OF LUNG — 1
CANCER OF STOMACH — .5
CANCER OF BREAST — 0.67
CANCER OF CERVIX — 0.33

PERSONS (0, 0.2, 0.4, 0.6, 0.8, 1.0)

All socioeconomic classes were included in the practice population, although there were somewhat more "middle class" people in it than there were in England and Wales as a whole for the same period. For roughly the first half of the period Fry was in solo practice; after that he had a partner. He devised and maintained careful and accurate records of each person's illnesses and visits.

Classifying the illnesses in the practice population into groups of diseases, he found the following distribution: respiratory illnesses 30 percent, emotional disorders 12 percent, gastrointestinal disorders 10 percent, skin disorders 10 percent, rheumatic disorders and disorders of the locomotor system 8 percent, cardiovascular and blood disorders 7.5 percent and all other disorders 22.5 percent. On the basis of his findings Fry calculated the annual morbidity experience in a typical British general practice of 2,500 people [see illustration at left]. Minor illnesses clearly predominate.

In summing up his experience Fry concluded that patients will seek medical care from the general practitioner for only about a fourth of all the illnesses that occur in the community. For the remainder they will accept the discomfort or handle the problem themselves by self-medication. Approximately two-thirds of the ailments that the physician does see in general practice are minor conditions that are self-limited, short in duration and unlikely to cause any permanent aftereffects. Major diseases, the potential killers, account for only about 5 percent of all illnesses. Even here there are qualifications. For example, two-thirds of the cases of hypertension were mild and merely involved elevated blood pressure without evidence of organ damage when they were discovered, and they required no specific treatment at all for years. The remaining third developed the symptoms and signs of hypertension and required treatment. With respect to cancer Fry points out that it is not a common disease, and that overall more than a third of the people with cancer survived for five years or longer regardless of therapy.

Considerable information regarding

ANNUAL MORBIDITY EXPERIENCE in a typical British general practice of 2,500 people is cited by the author as an example of how the ills of man are perceived by physicians. The data used to make this bar chart are based on observations made over a 17-year period by a British general practitioner, John Fry, and published in 1966 in his book *Profiles of Disease: A Study in the Natural History of Common Diseases.*

the true occurrence of illnesses, particularly minor illnesses, has been obtained by the careful observation and documentation of illness over a period of years in selected and defined populations by people themselves in collaboration with physicians. Such studies have the advantage of the highly accurate enumeration and characterization of illnesses, but they have the disadvantage of being limited to a small segment of the population. Thus they cannot be extrapolated to the population at large, except perhaps in a very general way.

An example is a 10-year study of a defined population of families in Cleveland carried out by the staff of the Department of Preventive Medicine at Western Reserve University School of Medicine from January, 1948, through May, 1957. The broad objectives were to determine as reliably as possible how much illness occurred, what its causes were, how important the family was in the spread of illness and how specific disease entities behaved as indicated by clinical, epidemiological and laboratory evidence.

The families included in this study constituted a carefully selected population chosen for stability in the community and for intelligent cooperation. The purposes and nature of the study were presented in detail to the prospective participants before they decided to collaborate. The families were presumably normal and were not selected because of illness in any member or because of either unusual frequency or absence of illness in the family unit. The parents of the families were young adults who had at least one child.

On admission of a family to the study the medical status of each member was determined by history, physical examination, chest X ray and examination of the blood and urine. Other types of examination such as electrocardiograms or blood-chemistry analyses were performed as indicated. A specimen of the blood was obtained as a basis of reference for later studies. Examinations were repeated at six-month intervals for children and annually for adults.

The data used in the analysis of illnesses came from records made as the illnesses appeared in each family. The mother was instructed in detail about record-keeping and notification of the department at the time of illness, however minor, in any individual in the household. At the beginning of each month the mother was given a new record sheet for each member of the family on which to note symptoms as they appeared on any date. Each family was visited weekly by a fieldworker or nurse

CLASS OF ILLNESS	NUMBER OF ILLNESSES	ILLNESSES PER PERSON-YEAR	PERCENT OF ALL ILLNESSES
TOTAL ILLNESSES	25,155	9.4	100
COMMON RESPIRATORY DISEASES	14,990	5.6	60
SPECIFIC RESPIRATORY DISEASES	793	0.3	3
INFECTIOUS GASTROENTERITIS	4,057	1.5	16
OTHER INFECTIONS	1,931	0.7	8
OTHER ILLNESSES	3,384	1.3	13

TEN-YEAR STUDY of a carefully selected, well-defined population of families in Cleveland was carried out from January, 1948, through May, 1957, by the author and his colleagues at the Western Reserve University School of Medicine. This summary of the results of that study provides an insight into yet another way of looking at the ills of man: as they are perceived by people themselves in close collaboration with physicians. Such studies are highly accurate in enumerating the incidence of major classes of illnesses, but so far they have been limited to small populations. During the 10-year duration of the Cleveland project a total of 86 families and 443 individuals were in the study at one time or another.

who reviewed the health status for the preceding week, discussed the mother's records with her and obtained a throat culture from each member of the household. Unless the complaint was trivial, every sick person was visited at the time of illness by a staff physician who recorded the clinical characteristics of the illness and the epidemiological circumstances surrounding it; the physician also obtained such specimens as were indicated for laboratory examination and arranged for other special tests when they were appropriate. The frequency of follow-up visits depended on the severity and duration of the illness. Patients who were hospitalized were seen in the hospital during the period of the acute illness. The records of the mothers, the fieldworkers and the staff physicians were reviewed regularly by members of the professional staff and a diagnosis was made for each illness. Such diagnoses were obviously attended by varying degrees of difficulty, some illnesses being recognized with a higher degree of reliability than others.

During the 10-year period a total of 86 families and 443 individuals were in the study at one time or another for a combined total of 970,036 person-days, 2,692 person-years or 556 family-years of observation. The population consisted of 172 parents, 138 male children and 133 female children. Eighty-four children were born into the study. The size of the families ranged from three to eight members, with the most common size being five. The median age of the parents at the time of entering the study was 30 for the mother and 33 for the father. At the time of entry the families were in the middle or upper economic groups. Except for short periods early in the study, each family lived by itself in

a single house and was regarded as an epidemiological unit. At the time of admission to the study the general medical status of the population was considered to be excellent and no one at that time had an incapacitating chronic disorder. As time went on various individuals developed abnormalities such as diabetes mellitus, multiple sclerosis, gout, otosclerosis and hypertension. No child developed rheumatic fever and no one had frank rheumatoid arthritis. Furthermore, no one experienced a myocardial infarction or angina pectoris, two common heart ailments. Malignant cancer was found in only one girl, who died of acute leukemia.

A total of 25,155 separate illnesses were diagnosed, which breaks down to a rate of 9.4 illnesses per person-year. The number of illnesses and average incidence rates for several broad diagnostic categories are shown in the illustration above. The term "common respiratory diseases," which was used to describe 60 percent of all illnesses, included the common cold, rhinitis, laryngitis, bronchitis and other acute respiratory illnesses of undifferentiated types. "Specific respiratory diseases" included streptococcal tonsillitis and pharyngitis, nonbacterial tonsillitis and pharyngitis, primary atypical pneumonia (mycoplasmal), pneumococcal pneumonia and influenza. Laboratory evidence was required for the diagnosis of streptococcal infection and influenza.

Infectious gastroenteritis, a disease of the intestinal tract, constituted the second most frequent group of illnesses encountered in this study. Clinical studies suggested that there were at least two types of gastroenteritis. One type was characterized by normal temperature, loss of appetite, nausea, abdominal pain

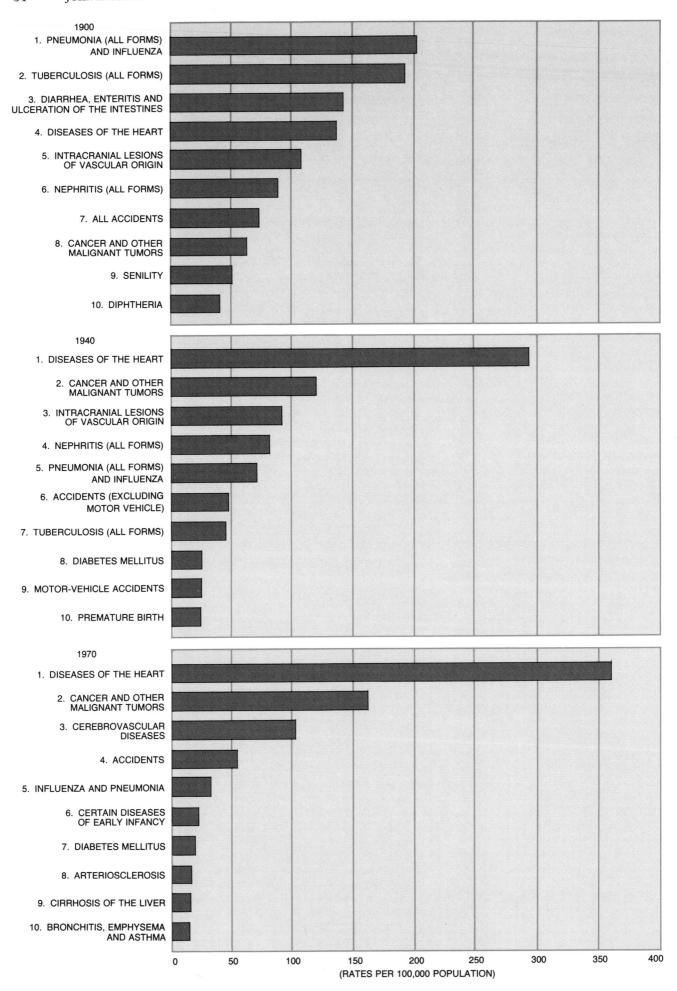

(RATES PER 100,000 POPULATION)

and diarrhea. The other type was characterized by fever, headache, nausea, vomiting, abdominal cramps and little or no diarrhea. When both types of gastroenteritis were transferred to volunteers, no cross-immunity could be demonstrated. The presumption therefore is that there are at least two types of acute viral gastroenteritis and that they are caused by different agents. The disease could not be transmitted to animals nor could any virus be isolated from either type.

"Other" infections included the usual diseases of childhood, otitis media (inflammation of the middle ear), viral infections of the herpes type and a miscellany of other illnesses, most of which were instances of unexplained fever without respiratory or intestinal symptoms or other evidence of localization. The category "Other illnesses" was made up of a variety of events, chiefly noninfectious.

Much more data of this kind could be presented from the Cleveland family study and from similar studies that have been carried out in the U.S. and in other countries in the past 15 years. Some of these studies have led to the isolation and identification of new viruses as causes of respiratory and other ailments in man. What is more to the point is the fact that people and physicians can combine and collaborate to present a reliable picture of the ills of man even though it is in a small and selected fragment of the population. Continued studies in segments of the population will slowly expand the picture to include the population as a whole.

For more than 100 years some countries have required the reporting of deaths and their causes (as far as they could be ascertained) to local and central authorities (usually public-health departments). The reporting of the fact of death is highly reliable since apart from unusual homicides there is little reluctance to give such notification. Causes of

VITAL STATISTICS provide an additional vantage point for perceiving and classifying the ills of man. The bar charts on the opposite page, for example, list the 10 leading causes of death in the U.S. for the years 1900, 1940 and 1970 in order of decreasing death rates. Certain changes in terminology occurred during this interval. For example, "intracranial lesions of vascular origin" (1940) correspond to "cerebrovascular diseases" (1970). Concurrently with the changes depicted in this illustration the average life expectancy at birth in the U.S. increased from 47 years in 1900 to 71 in 1970.

death are less accurately reported and frequently cannot be determined with assurance. Legal requirements for the reporting of "notifiable" diseases, which are almost entirely infectious and communicable in character, vary from state to state in the U.S. Since 1928 all the states have submitted reports at least annually to the Public Health Service. The completeness and accuracy of the reporting varies with the nature and severity of the disease and with the conscientiousness of whatever physicians attend the patient. Measles, for example, is poorly reported because it is rarely very serious or fatal, and most cases are not even seen by a physician. In contrast, the potentially more dangerous diseases, such as diphtheria, smallpox and typhoid, if they are recognized as such, are usually reported.

From data such as these and associated demographic information the compiler of vital statistics composes his picture of the ills of man. Even though he never sees a patient, his picture is not to be deprecated, since many important inferences can be drawn from it to aid evaluators and planners not only in the health field but also in other social and economic enterprises. Moreover, the consideration of changes in the past can help in estimating the possibilities of future developments.

For example, the 10 leading causes of death in the U.S. for the years 1900, 1940 and 1970 are listed in the illustration on the opposite page in order of decreasing rates of death. Expansion of the registration areas to include all the states and some changes in the definition of causes of death occurred in this 71-year period, but for our purposes we may consider that the appropriate categories are similar in composition; for example, "intracranial lesions of vascular origin" (1940) correspond to "cerebrovascular diseases" (1970). In 1900 the three leading causes of death were infectious and communicable diseases (pneumonia/influenza, tuberculosis, and diarrhea/enteritis). The 10 leading causes of death also included diphtheria and nephritis (for the most part postinfectious).

In the next 40 years there were major changes. Three noninfectious diseases became the three top causes of death: heart disease, cancer and intracranial lesions of vascular origin. Heart disease and cancer showed a marked increase; pneumonia and tuberculosis showed equally dramatic decreases.

By 1970 the noninfectious diseases, particularly the diseases of aging, became even more prominent. Tuberculosis disappeared from the list, and influenza and pneumonia comprised the only

remaining category of infectious and communicable diseases.

Concurrently with the change during the 71-year period the average life expectancy at birth increased from 47 years in 1900 to 71 in 1970. The average length of life for females exceeded that of males by two years in 1900 and eight years in 1970. Part of the increase in the average life expectancy of females and the increasing difference between females and males are apparently due to the decline in maternal mortality rates (deaths from natural causes per 100,000 live births) from 607.9 in 1915 to an estimated 27.4 in 1970.

The reasons for the dramatic increase in life expectancy and changes in the major causes of death are multiple, overlapping and complex and have never been sharply delineated. Moreover, they seem to have begun slowly in the middle of the 19th century after the disruptions resulting from the Industrial Revolution had begun to diminish and long before any specific prophylaxis and therapy were available. Included among the responsible factors were improvements in environmental sanitation, particularly water purification and sewage disposal, and better housing, clothing and nutrition. One factor that was and still is of major importance is the decline in the incidence and lethality of the infectious and communicable diseases of infancy and childhood, including tuberculosis. I shall briefly cite three examples.

The mortality rate from tuberculosis in Europe and North America was estimated to be approximately 500 per 100,000 people per year in the middle of the 19th century. By 1900 the death rate in the U.S. had fallen to slightly less than 200 deaths per 100,000 people per year. Thereafter there was a strong, steady decline to a rate of 2.8 in 1969. There was a similar decline in the death rate from typhoid fever [*see illustration on next page*]. No immunization against tuberculosis has been adopted in the U.S., and the effectiveness of typhoid vaccine is questionable. Immunization against diphtheria, however, has probably been an important factor in the decline in the incidence and mortality of the disease, although the case-fatality ratio (expressed as the percentage of recognized cases that die irrespective of treatment) has remained relatively constant for the past 50 years. This fact suggests that there has been little change in the basic lethality of the disease.

Although general factors associated with improved standards of living have undoubtedly contributed to the decline in the incidence and mortality of the

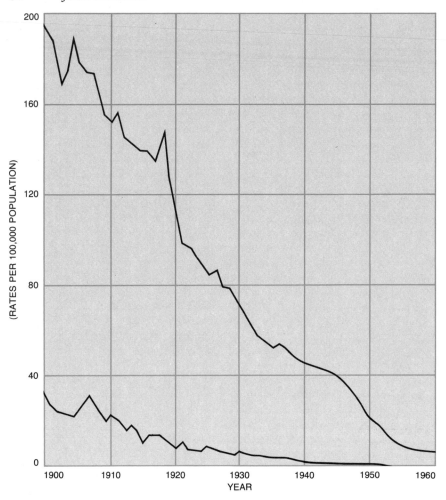

(RATES PER 100,000 POPULATION)

YEAR

DECLINING DEATH RATES attributable to the infectious and communicable diseases of infancy and childhood, such as tuberculosis (*upper curve*) and typhoid fever (*lower curve*), are a major factor in the dramatic increase in life expectancy in the U.S. in this century. General factors associated with improved standards of living have contributed greatly to the decline in the incidence and the mortality of such diseases, although specific public-health measures have also been important. No immunization against tuberculosis has been adopted in the U.S., and the effectiveness of typhoid vaccine is questionable.

communicable diseases of childhood, other specific measures have also been important. Among them are the eradication of tuberculous cattle, the various activities of health officers in health education and in case finding and follow-up, immunization campaigns to augment natural resistance and "herd" immunity and, in the past 40 years, the discovery of many effective chemotherapeutic and antibiotic drugs. The gain has been increased longevity; the cost has been the increase in chronic and degenerative diseases associated with aging.

The ills of man have been considered in this article from the perspective of people themselves, of physicians, of people in close collaboration with physicians and of keepers of vital statistics. From all four viewpoints the chief burden of man's ailments, numerically at least, consists of acute, benign, self-limited illnesses. As longevity increases, however, the chronic degenerative diseases rapidly come to dominate the causes of death and disability. Many other perspectives exist, such as the viewpoint of the environmentalist and his concern with the ills resulting from pollution, and the viewpoint of those concerned with mental illness.

Much can be done to prevent and alleviate illness, but death is inevitable; in the final analysis the death rate is 100 percent. As René J. Dubos has written (in his book *Mirage of Health*): "Life is an adventure where nothing is static.... Every manifestation of existence is a response to stimuli and challenge, each of which constitutes a threat if not adequately dealt with. The very process of living is a continual interplay between the individual and his environment, often taking the form of a struggle resulting in injury or disease.... Complete and lasting freedom from disease is but a dream."

VI

Surgical Intervention

albule oculōs sic excutiunt

fungus de nare
sic inciditur:

Surgical Intervention

CHARLES G. CHILD III

Man intervenes in his ills with surgery, with chemical methods and with psychiatry. Surgery can win heroic victories, but its everyday practice calls for the control of quantity and quality

Surgery, for most people, is the word for crucial intervention to change the course of serious disease. It is not necessarily so, of course; there are many small operations and diagnostic procedures and there are large areas in which chemical, psychological and other kinds of medical intervention can play at least as critical a role in therapy. Yet surgery remains one of the most explicit and, for better and for worse, the most dramatic form of intervention. And it constitutes a major part of the country's health system. Between 40,000 and 50,-000 major and minor operations are performed every day in the 5,770 U.S. hospitals with surgical facilities; about half of those hospitals' beds are occupied by surgical patients and more than a third of the patients discharged from them every day have undergone an operation.

Contemporary American surgery is very good indeed—probably the best in the world. It could be better, however. In this article I shall not dwell much on the advances in training, scientific investigation and technique that make surgery at its best so effective; rather I shall concentrate on issues that trouble me and some of my colleagues as we consider the ability of our specialties to measure up to their potential. Many of these issues involve what may be called quality control and· accountability: the need to measure, evaluate and improve the degree of excellence achieved by individual surgeons, the hospitals in which they work and the operations they undertake to perform.

Surgery is a healing art that seeks to alleviate human suffering and prolong people's lives. It cannot logically be removed from the rest of modern medicine, since it is only one therapy, fitted as required into the overall management of sick people; a surgeon is "a doctor who can operate." The surgeon's work requires a large number of intellectual, mechanical and manual dexterities. His tools include (in addition to a lively and thoughtful understanding of his discipline) knives, scissors, hemostats, cauteries, ligatures, needles, X rays, ultrasound and lasers; prostheses made of fabrics, metals and plastics; clips, nails and screws. With the aid of this array of tools he makes bold to invade almost all the body's tissues, organs and cavities, repairing, removing and replacing. By today's standards these activities were once uncomplicated and direct; now they have become hugely sophisticated and complex—and accurate. Once speed was of the essence; the development of anesthesia made that less important, and now improved methods of anesthesia mean that time can be taken to ensure precision, care and thoroughness in any procedure.

Some of surgery is exciting and even dramatic; all of it is highly visible. A great deal of it is plain hard work, often repetitive. It is essentially a team activity; surgeons, anesthesiologists, radiologists, nurses, technicians, ward maids and orderlies are inseparably responsible, and the entire team must be available around the clock (even though something less than 10 percent of surgery is an emergency matter). By its very nature surgery is emotionally demanding for the patient, his family and the operating team. This is in part because the result of surgery is generally less equivocal than that of some other kinds of intervention. When the result is good, the surgeon is likely to be considered a hero. By the same token it is easy to make him a villain, so that malpractice-insurance premiums are several times higher for surgeons than they are for internists, pediatricians or psychiatrists. Obviously surgery does not cure everyone, and by its very nature it may often be the culminating event of a terminal illness or a fatal accident.

There are two things everyone knows about surgery today. It is specialized and it is expensive. As to specialization, the human body has been subdivided into precise domains, with each claim staked out and jealously guarded by surgeons, specialty boards, hospitals and even knowing patients; the complaint is often made that such specialization (as in other fields of medicine) results in treatment of a condition rather than a patient. It is clear, however, that the time is long since past when a surgeon could learn and practice every known surgical procedure. There are simply too many procedures; one of the most useful current classifications of surgical interventions lists almost 1,000. And so the "general surgeon" now confines his efforts to the

SURGERY OF THE EYE AND THE NOSE is portrayed in the engraving on the opposite page, which dates from the 12th century. The Latin caption of the top drawing reads: "Cataracts of the eyes are cut out thus." The surgeon is probably about to "couch" a cataract, penetrating the eye with a needle and turning the clouded lens down out of the line of sight. The patient holds an ointment jar. The lower drawing is captioned: "A polyp is cut from the nose thus." The patient holds a bowl for catching blood. These drawings, several versions of which are found in medieval medical-surgical handbooks, are from the herbal of Dioscorides, derived from *De Materia Medica*, and also prepared by the Greek physician Dioscorides in the first century. It is one of the Harley Manuscripts in the British Museum.

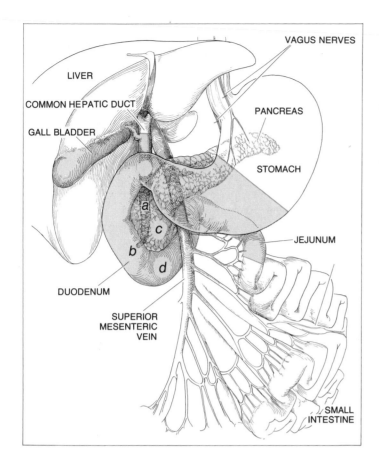

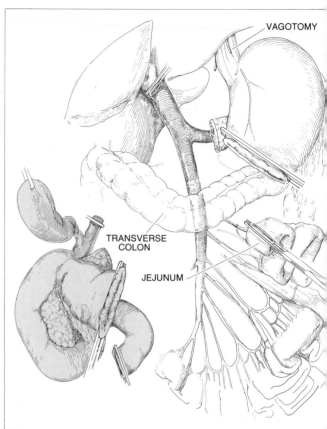

PANCREATICODUODENECTOMY is an extensive operation that primarily involves removal of the duodenum (the first segment of the small intestine) and about half of the stomach and the pancreas and reconstruction of the digestive tract. The extent of the operation is shown (*color*) at left, along with the sites of origin of the cancers for which it is appropriate: the common bile duct (*a*); the papilla of Vater (*b*), where the bile and pancreatic ducts enter the duodenum; the head of the pancreas (*c*); the duodenum (*d*).

abdomen and perhaps a few other organs unclaimed by other specialists. Neurosurgeons deal with the brain, spinal cord and nerves, thoracic surgeons with the contents of the chest, orthopedists with the bones and joints. Gynecologists, urologists, ophthalmologists, otolaryngologists and others each operate on their respective organs and tissues. (Each specialty has its own triumphs and shortcomings, of which its practitioners are uniquely conscious; it is surely presumptuous for one surgeon to speak in this article for the entire field, but the nature of this issue of *Scientific American* and of this article has made that necessary.)

As for expense, there are a few things that should be said, although the problem is essentially one that pervades all medical services and is dealt with at greater length in other articles in this issue [see "The Hospital," by John H. Knowles, page 91, and "The Medical Economy," by Martin Feldstein, page 112]. The bulk of the cost of surgery is the cost of hospital care. I recently operated on a man with cancer of the duodenum, more specifically, cancer of the papilla of Vater [see *illustration above*]. He was elderly and not a particularly good risk; laboratory tests substantiated a clear history of heart disease. He required many days of preoperative preparation and then of postoperative treatment in the intensive-care unit to protect him during recovery. He was in the hospital for 35 days and received a bill for $13,488. (Needless to say, if he had had only a hernia repaired, his hospital bill would have been much smaller. If, on the other hand, his stay had been complicated by lung, heart or kidney failure, his bill could have been much larger. And he might have died.)

My patient is home now; his cancer was small, without evidence of spreading, and he has probably been cured. Having undertaken to treat him on the traditional fee-for-service basis, what should I charge for his operation? I turn to Blue Shield of Michigan for advice and learn that "the range of charges for pancreatectomy, subtotal, Whipple-type is $500 to $1,325." What is fair—to me, to the patient, to society?

Surgery appears to lend itself particularly well to fee-for-service payment: it is a discrete event, a service rendered; why should not the surgeon be paid for his work? As a nonmedical admirer of American medicine has written, "Like any other small entrepreneur, the solo practitioner lives or dies economically by how well he satisfies his customers." And yet the fee for service is difficult to defend. If the patient is paying, it puts a burden on low-income patients or requires charity on the part of the surgeon. If an insurance carrier is paying, the system limits the surgeon to an arbitrary and often capricious set of fees and makes no distinction among surgeons of differing quality. The system also puts pressure on the surgeon to operate as much as possible. (If he is ethical and careful, he will not operate unnecessarily, but he may work himself to death.) In the face of all these disadvantages, the fact remains that it is not easy to design a completely satisfactory alternative to the fee for service. And yet I suspect that alternative systems will be in wide use before long. (Such systems should cope, incidentally, with the problem of what surgeons should charge for not operating

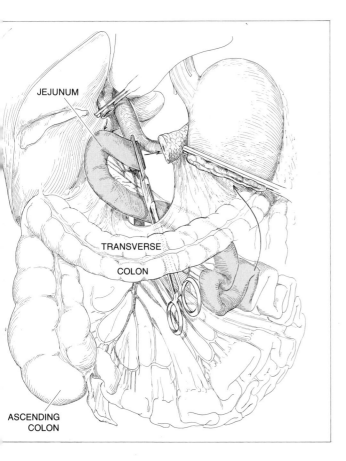

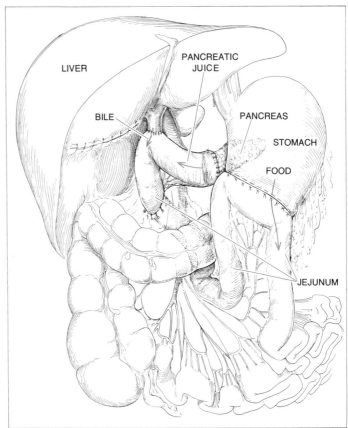

After exploratory maneuvers to determine the resectability of the cancer, the tissues to be excised (*color*) are removed (*second from left*). In order to reconstitute the digestive tract a length of jejunum (*color*), the next segment of the intestine, is approximated (*black arrows*) to the bile duct, the remaining pancreas and the stomach (*third from left*). Thereafter end-to-end and end-to-side connections are made (*right*). Reconstruction of digestive tract shown in the drawings is compatible with normal digestion (*colored arrows*).

on a patient. Not to operate involves decisions that may well require as much training and judgment and consideration as operating.)

Closely related to the expense of surgery is the question of its availability. The general public believes that medical manpower and resources are in short supply. Most thoughtful professionals are more likely to believe that total resources are adequate and that the real problems are those of distribution and quality. There are indications that advanced surgical skills are actually underutilized. One study shows that even if all operations were done by specialists, their average work load would be fewer than five operations a week, far below capacity.

As for facilities, the consensus is that the total number of hospital beds available for surgical patients is adequate or even too large. Still, the relation between supply and demand is a tricky one. Consider the case of kidney transplantation. In 1971, 1,610 patients received transplants, even though it has been estimated that some 5,000 victims of kidney disease die every year who

could be saved by a transplant. The procedure is terribly expensive, however, and the cost has been the barrier between this form of treatment and the patients who need it. Now Congress has passed a law providing Medicare reimbursement for kidney transplantation (or artificial-kidney treatment) for any patient with end-stage kidney disease. Now there will (quite rightly) be no financial bar to the therapy, and so new problems will be exposed: a serious lack of specialized facilities and trained personnel—and of kidneys. Moreover, as good as the law is for patients with advanced kidney disease, it fails to provide for a host of other ills quite as catastrophic. The propriety of a law that discriminates in favor of a single class of patients has been questioned by many legislators and physicians. Shortages similar to those revealed by the kidney-disease legislation will become apparent as the country finally faces up to the broader problem of making medical care available to everyone as a right.

Assuming that what people have a right to is not minimal care or mediocre care but good care, questions of quality arise: Is the surgeon skillful and are the other personnel well trained? Is the operating room clean and properly equipped? Is the operation justified? Was the preoperative work-up thorough? Does it all go smoothly and safely? The patient and his family assume that the answers are all yes. Medical professionals like to assume the same thing, but many of them know that it is not always so.

Who are surgeons, first of all, and by what sanctions, public or private, do they presume to cut into living tissue? Once they were shamans, or priests; then they were barbers; in this country even during most of the 19th century they were self-taught and self-anointed. Things are different now, but the transition from do-it-yourself training and qualification to licensing and certification took more than 100 years. Surgeons follow their profession today under what is still an amalgam of private, voluntary and public sanctions, the basis of which is the American tradition that a profession regulates itself. It is only in the past few years, as the Federal Government gets increasingly into the business of paying for health care, that the Government has set standards. For the most part it has taken over and written into law the standards of private and voluntary agencies.

States license surgeons to practice. States also license the hospitals where operations take place. Society has demanded more protection than that, however, and so a host of private and voluntary nonprofit boards, commissions, associations and committees have come into the picture, mostly without legal authorization but with varying degrees of effectiveness. During the early part of this century surgeons realized that licensure was a minimal qualification. One by one each surgical specialty generated a board that would prescribe the length and content of training beyond medical school, identify the hospitals where it could take place and examine and certify candidates as specialists. The first such board was formed in 1916 for ophthalmology, a field then plagued by quackery. Others followed. The American Board of Surgery was established in 1937 to certify the general surgeon. Even today, however, many surgeons are not board-certified [*see top illustration on page 66*]. Anyone who has been licensed can declare himself a specialist in an exotic surgical procedure and operate—provided he can find a hospital that will let him.

As a matter of fact sick people in the U.S. are quite literally at the mercy of the regulations and practices of whatever hospital they find themselves in. That makes hospital accreditation important, to say the least. Accreditation is the province of another private entity, the Joint Commission on Accreditation of Hospitals, which was established in 1952 by the American Medical Association, the colleges of physicians and of surgeons and the American Hospital Association. It surveys almost all hospitals with more than 100 beds, some 75 percent of those with between 50 and 100 beds and a few of the smaller, mostly private hospitals. To be accredited a hospital must meet standards as to equipment, housekeeping, regulations and certain procedures, such as adequate review of all operations. It need not, however, require that all operations be performed by specialists, and the commission has been criticized for that. In any case accreditation has now been grafted into Federal legislation: the Medicare amendment to the Social Security Act in 1965 provides that in order to qualify for Medicare payments a hospital must meet standards set by the Secretary of Health, Education, and Welfare—but that these requirements may not be higher than those established by the commission. In effect, a commission-accredited hospital qualifies for Medicare.

Is that the way it should be done? This newly focused question of how to coordinate public and private standards is not an easy one, and it tends to draw

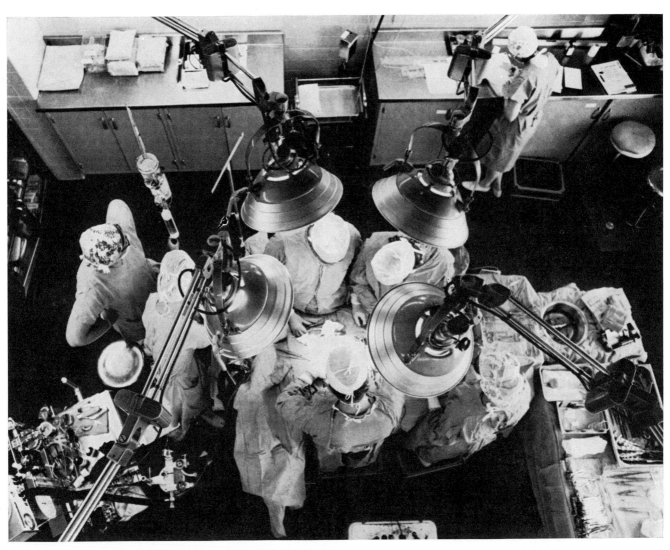

ABDOMINAL OPERATION is performed at Children's Hospital in Boston in one of the eight operating rooms in the 330-bed hospital, which is affiliated with the Harvard Medical School. The picture was made from a viewing gallery above a glass skylight.

physicians and legislators into a polite contest. The physicians try to impress their standards on government, whereas politicians and administrators question the propriety of writing into public law professional rules that have been written by nonpublic bodies. In 1969 the Health Insurance Benefits Advisory Council reported to the Secretary of Health, Education, and Welfare that it seemed "inappropriate" to delegate all Government authority to safeguard the quality of medical care to "a private agency."

Yet that may be the only way to get standards into law. Two of Medicare's stillborn predecessors, the Forand bills of 1957 and 1959, stipulated that reimbursement would be made only to a surgeon who was certified by the American Board of Surgery or was a member of the American College of Surgeons. The bills were never passed. And when Medicare was enacted in 1965, the legislation defined "physician" as any "doctor of medicine or osteopathy legally au-

thorized to practice medicine and surgery by the state." Now, I am not so naïve as to believe that the Forand bills failed simply because they stipulated that only recognized specialists would receive public money. I guess I am sophisticated enough, however, to recognize that the proposed discrimination among practicing surgeons, many of whom were not certified, did not make friends for the bills among uncertified surgeons. Too many of them were making too much money practicing as self-declared specialists or as "general practitioner" surgeons. I can also appreciate the fact that adopting private professional standards as the basis for the payment of public funds could create legislative and judicial problems. Moreover, medical licensing is a state function, so that the Federal standards proposed in the Forand bills might have seemed to be an invasion of states' rights. Whatever the reasons, we now have the Medicare legislation, and it does not do what

it might have done: protect patients by ensuring that surgical operations (except for emergencies) must be performed by people precisely qualified to perform them.

Such protection is needed, and for the foreseeable future it will have to be achieved by a combination of public and private standards. I suspect that as time passes the Government is going to have more to say about it. These problems have been more easily solved in some other countries with more government domination of medicine. In Sweden hospitals are run by county governments and surgeons are employed by those governments. A Swedish physician who finds much to criticize in his country's system nevertheless writes that "nowhere in Sweden will a major surgical procedure be done by an unqualified surgeon." In Britain much the same situation applies, with all hospitals run by the central government. In Canada the Royal College of Physicians and Sur-

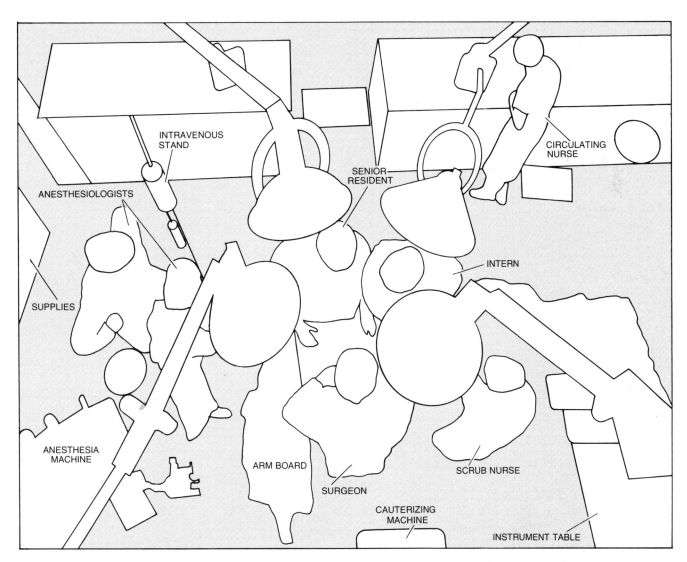

PERSONNEL AND EQUIPMENT in the photograph on the opposite page are identified. The surgeon is assisted by a resident and an intern. The anesthesiologist is responsible for monitoring the patient's vital signs as well as for administering the anesthetic itself.

geons was established in 1929 by an act of Parliament. It approves hospitals and sets common nationwide standards and examinations for physicians' and surgeons' credentials. Moreover, Canadian hospitals are paid by insurance systems operated by the provincial governments; surgeons who are not certified are not likely to be paid specialists' rates.

Surgeons, patients and the public at large all recognize that some kind of ratio of success to failure is at least one important index of the quality of an individual surgeon, of a specific procedure or method, of a hospital or hospital system or of the total national delivery of surgical care. Creating such indexes is not easy. Professional journals are filled with reports of survival rates, cures, complications and deaths, but it is dangerous and unsatisfactory to project these to the population as a whole. Some kind of overall evaluation is nonetheless necessary.

To begin with, what is surgical success or failure? Success may be quite simple: if an appendix is removed for acute appendicitis, the patient will be cured and will never have appendicitis again. The outcome is more complex even in the case of hernias: they can recur and require another operation. In cancer or open-heart surgery or kidney transplantation the result may not be clear for many years: cancers can recur, mechanical heart valves can fail, a kidney can be rejected. As for surgical failure, one obvious measure is the incidence of fatal outcomes or life-threatening complications. This is a tricky business, however, and the raw figures can be misleading.

If in a certain hospital no surgery is conducted, there will be no surgical mortality at all. If in another hospital operations are performed but the staff is overcautious and accepts only very good risks as patients, the mortality figures may be very low. There are hospitals, however, whose staffs are more courageous and, given the proper indications, accept almost all comers for surgical intervention; their mortality may be sub-

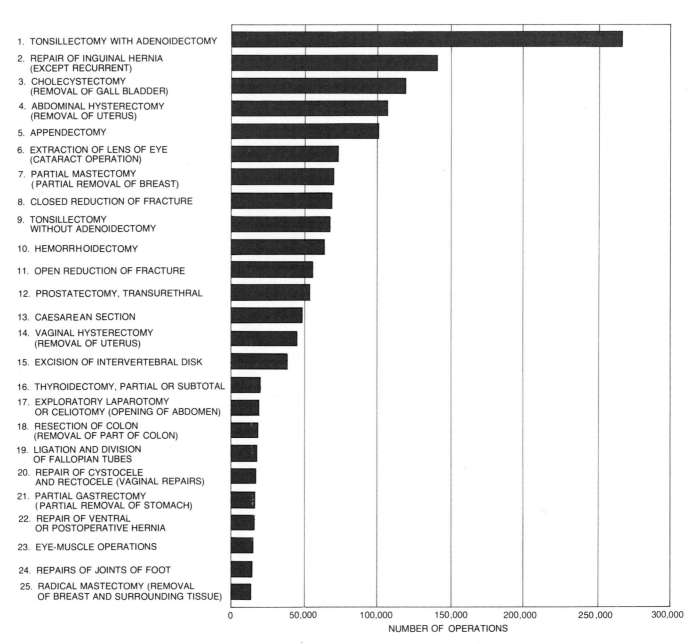

TWENTY-FIVE MOST FREQUENT OPERATIONS of appreciable magnitude being performed are these. The list is based on a tabulation, by the Professional Activity Study of the Commission on Professional and Hospital Activities, of the 50 operations done most often (as most important operation) in 1969, from which diagnostic procedures and those of small scope were eliminated.

stantially higher. Clearly mortality rates have to be considered with due regard for patient populations as well as procedures. (On the other hand, if there is a hospital where most patients die after operations, it is pretty safe to say that the hospital should be closed down.)

Given these qualifying considerations, the fact remains that postoperative mortality is a most important statistic for assessing surgical quality. It is only recently that we have even begun to collect the necessary numbers on a national scale. First of all, what operations are being performed? Every year the Professional Activity Study of the Commission on Professional and Hospital Activities records the 50 most frequent operations in its member hospitals, which treat about a third of the patients in the country's non-Federal short-term hospitals. I have taken the 1969 survey's tabulation and removed from it the procedures that are primarily diagnostic and those of small scope in order to prepare a list of the 25 most frequent surgical interventions of appreciable magnitude [*see illustration on opposite page*].

Now let us consider the postoperative mortality associated with 11 of these procedures, which I have selected somewhat arbitrarily to illustrate the full range. The mortality figures are for hospitals covered by the Professional Activity Study in 1969 [*see illustration above*]. The lowest mortality, only .3 per 10,000 operations, was for tonsillectomy without adenoidectomy. The highest mortality, 1,328 per 10,000, was for exploratory laparotomy or celiotomy (opening of the abdomen). It should be noted that no assumption can be made about the actual cause of death; these are simply the postoperative death rates associated with each procedure.

How should one read a mortality table of this kind? Here are a few thoughts on just some of the procedures listed:

Ligation and division of the Fallopian tubes ("tying the tubes" that lead from the ovaries to the uterus) is a sterilization procedure. The operation has a low death rate. Is one death per 20,000 operations acceptable in terms of population control and individual family planning? Most people seem to believe it is.

Many abdominal hysterectomies, or removals of the uterus, are legitimate procedures intended to remedy an identified disease. Some—an unknown number—are nonetheless performed without clear surgical indications. The death rate is not negligible, and if the mortality is acceptable when the operation is justi-

OPERATION	NUMBER OF OPERATIONS	NUMBER OF DEATHS	DEATHS PER 10,000 OPERATIONS
TONSILLECTOMY WITHOUT ADENOIDECTOMY	68,127	2	.3
LIGATION AND DIVISION OF FALLOPIAN TUBES	18,195	1	.5
PARTIAL MASTECTOMY	70,692	52	7.4
ABDOMINAL HYSTERECTOMY	107,860	220	20.4
APPENDECTOMY	100,946	355	35.2
RADICAL MASTECTOMY	15,119	61	40.3
PROSTATECTOMY, TRANSURETHRAL	54,413	893	164.1
OPEN REDUCTION OF FRACTURE	56,343	2,672	474.2
PARTIAL GASTRECTOMY	16,834	975	579.2
RESECTION OF COLON	18,975	1,607	846.9
EXPLORATORY LAPAROTOMY OR CELIOTOMY	19,139	2,542	1,328.2

POSTOPERATIVE MORTALITY, shown here for 1969 for 11 of the operations performed most frequently, varies widely with the nature of the operative procedure and the patients.

fied medically, it is certainly quite unacceptable when the operation is performed unnecessarily.

Appendectomy is generally accepted as a necessary and rather safe operation. One ought, however, to differentiate among appendectomies. The death rate in operations performed in 1969 for acute appendicitis without peritonitis was nine per 10,000; for appendicitis associated with peritonitis, the rate was 174 per 10,000. About a tenth of all appendectomies, however, are done for "other" appendicitis, and that is the controversial area. A number of those operations are probably unnecessary. Yet the death rate for this dubious category is fairly low: seven per 10,000. (After all, the patient is often quite healthy!) Perhaps one can argue that the public can afford to have some appendixes removed unnecessarily for "acute remunerative appendicitis" by less than scrupulous surgeons. Most people are happy to be rid of their appendix.

The highest death rate, 13 percent for exploration of the abdomen, is not hard to understand. Most of these operations are done on patients with some intra-abdominal catastrophe or with undiagnosed abdominal cancers, largely in order to see if something can perhaps be done surgically to relieve suffering or prolong life. The procedure is sometimes little more than the last rite of a terminal illness (in which case its economic justification ought perhaps to be questioned). On the other hand, in some cases the in-

vestigation establishes an important diagnosis that converts a bleak outlook into a hopeful prognosis or even a cure.

What is most disturbing, of course, is not that some operations are associated with a high mortality but that the mortality varies from hospital to hospital of roughly equivalent status. Five years ago Lincoln E. Moses of Stanford University and Frederick Mosteller of Harvard University did a study of almost 200,000 operations performed in 35 medical centers. They found differences in crude death rates as high as thirty- or fortyfold. When the figures were corrected for age, the seriousness of the condition and all other measurable variables, the death rates were still four or five times higher in some institutions than in others. A major attempt to analyze further such institutional differences in death rates is now being conducted at Stanford University under the auspices of the National Research Council.

Meanwhile the American Surgical Association and the American College of Surgeons are making a joint study of surgical services in the U.S. One objective is to find out how many surgical deaths and life-threatening complications are preventable. If the study concludes that only a tiny fraction might have been prevented, surgeons and hospitals will be able to relax, reassured that U.S. surgery truly is the best in the world. It is possible, however, that an honest and competent review will disclose that a substantial number of deaths and compli-

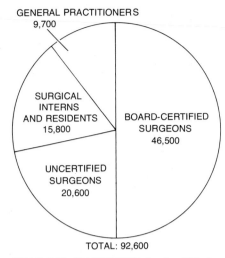

GENERAL PRACTITIONERS
9,700

SURGICAL
INTERNS
AND RESIDENTS
15,800

BOARD-CERTIFIED
SURGEONS
46,500

UNCERTIFIED
SURGEONS
20,600

TOTAL: 92,600

SURGICAL MANPOWER in the U.S. includes surgeons, general practitioners who operate, interns and residents. About two-thirds of the surgeons have been certified as surgeons; the others are self-designated.

cations could have been avoided—if the surgeon had been better trained, if he had exercised better judgment, if he had had better facilities. Such a finding would confront American surgeons and surgery with a definable crisis of credibility and of confidence.

Changing conditions and attitudes make it clear that surgery is approaching the status of a public utility. As dehumanizing as it may seem, surgeons are the providers and patients the consumers; hospitals are the facilities and insurance carriers or governments are the fiscal agents. (Everyone is a potential consumer; only the dead are immune from surgery and today even they are called on to provide spare parts for the living.) Public utilities have got to be accountable to the public, and account-

ability requires a very clear judgment of performance. Studies such as those I have mentioned will help, and so would a real improvement in the routine reporting of cause of death on death certificates. It seems to me, however, that the most direct way to measure the quality of surgery would be to establish a national registry to which every operation performed in the country would be reported: patient, diagnosis, operation, surgeon, hospital, outcome. Peer judgments regarding the operation should be included: Was it necessary? If there was a death or a life-threatening complication, could it have been avoided? If it was avoidable, was it the fault of the hospital, the surgeon, the community, the disease process or the stage of disease? Providing these data to the registry could be made a condition of licensure or specialty certification for surgeons and a condition of accreditation for hospitals.

Storage, retrieval and analysis of the data by computer should not be difficult; the cost would be great but would be trivial compared with that of moon walks or laboratories in the sky. At first, perhaps, the results should be utilized in the aggregate, for an overview of U.S. surgery's performance. Later, as surgeons and hospitals become adjusted to the idea, the reports could be made specific. Areas of excellence could be identified and maintained, mediocre surgery could be improved and bad surgery could be eliminated under law. At long last the country would have the information with which to repair some of the defects in the current system of delivering surgical care.

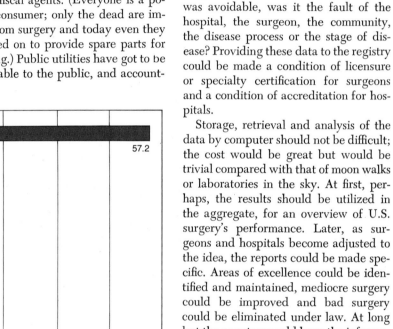

SURGICAL   57.2
ORTHOPEDIC   (19.0)
OBSTETRICAL AND
GYNECOLOGICAL   (15.4)
GASTROINTESTINAL   (11.5)
OTHER SURGICAL   (11.3)
MEDICAL   20.5
RADIOLOGICAL   6.1
EMERGENCY   5.8
ALL OTHERS   10.4

0   10   20   30   40   50   60
CLAIMS BY TYPE OF TREATMENT (PERCENT OF TOTAL)

MOST MALPRACTICE CLAIMS arise from surgical procedures, and in particular orthopedic surgery. The physicians most at risk are orthopedic surgeons and anesthesiologists.

VII

Chemical Intervention

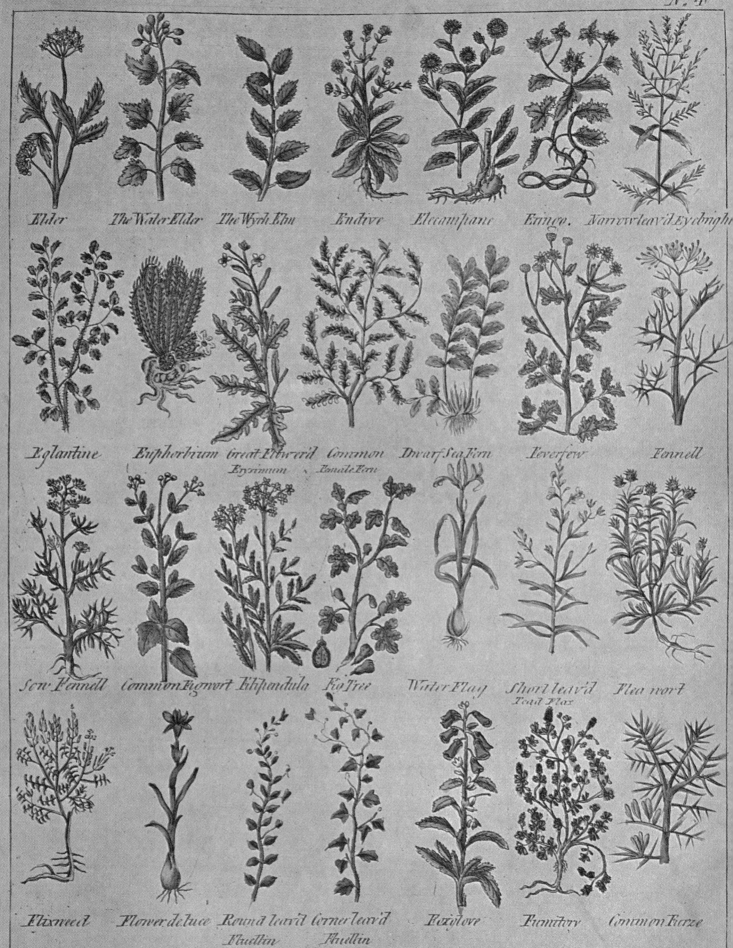

Elder The Water Elder The Wych Elm Endive Elecampane Esincy. Narrow leav'd Eyebright

Eglantine Euphorbium Great Flower'd Common Dwarf Sea Fern Feverfew Fennell
Erysimum Female Fern

Sow Fennell Common Figwort Filipendula Fig Tree Water Flag Short leav'd Flea wort
Toad Flax

Flixweed Flower de luce Round leav'd Corne leav'd Foxglove Fumitory Common Furze
Fluellin Fluellin

Publish'd as the Act Directs.

Chemical Intervention

SHERMAN M. MELLINKOFF

The chemical substances administered for medical purposes include not only drugs but also vaccines, hormones, anesthetics and even foods. All such measures lend themselves to use, abuse and misuse

A medical student asks: "Why is it that most of the drugs we prescribe are destroyed in the liver? How could nature have designed the liver to destroy drugs manufactured by man millions of years later?" The answer lies in the still dimly perceived universe of chemical reactions embodied in all living organisms. In those organisms that eat, food must be turned into the chemicals of life. The liver plays a key role in this extraordinary performance. Most of the blood that leaves the stomach and the intestines must pass through the liver before reaching the rest of the body. The liver is thus strategically placed to process nutrients and to detoxify poisons that might be ingested with the food.

It is therefore not surprising that when a chemist manufactures a drug, which somehow must alter the chemistry of the patient, the general structure of the new chemical has already been anticipated by the liver. The chemical structure of a refined drug is often similar to a naturally occurring substance. For example, alkaloids such as opium, from which heroin is derived, flourished in poppy plants that preceded man on the earth. Detoxification of such chemicals in the liver

can be regarded as one of the developments that enabled the species to survive. In the Garden of Eden the liver must have protected Adam from alkaloids, if not from the apple.

This relation between drugs and the liver illustrates two general aspects of man's chemical intervention in his own physiology. The first aspect is that life itself is an awe-inspiring multitude of natural chemical reactions. Sir Macfarlane Burnet put it succinctly: "It is very humbling to realize that there is more information packed into the head of one spermatozoon than there is in all the volumes of the *Journal of Biochemistry*." The second aspect is that when man deliberately alters these reactions, whether through chemicals derived from nature or through those manufactured by man in imitation of nature, there is a simultaneous potential for healing and for injury, sometimes for life or for death.

It is small wonder, then, that in man's ancient and even recent efforts at chemical intervention the health benefits have been far outweighed by chemical mayhem. In past centuries harmful agents were often prescribed by physicians (a little arsenic as a tonic) or imbibed unwittingly (lead in the wine goblets and

cooking utensils of ancient Rome). Destruction has been and still is sought out recklessly by some in opium or heroin addiction. Oliver Wendell Holmes was largely correct when he observed that "if all the drugs in the pharmacopoeia save three were dumped into the ocean, it would be so much the better for our patients and so much the worse for the fish." At the beginning of the 20th century there were only about six reliable and effective pharmaceutical preparations, namely digitalis (still helpful in many kinds of heart disease), morphine, quinine (for malaria), diphtheria antitoxin, aspirin and ether. Two other successful means of chemical intervention were also available: immunization against smallpox and rabies. This pharmacopoeia remained basically unchanged until about the time of World War II. Since then drugs and other substances that can, if employed wisely, usefully affect the chemistry of life have been produced in startling numbers.

The food we eat provides the chemicals the body needs to continue functioning. Much remains to be learned about what constitutes an optimal diet. Except where food intake is affected by peculiar food customs, by poverty, by social upheavals such as war, by drug addiction, by alcoholism or by some other illness, the nutrition of man today is generally much better than it was at any time in the past. It is difficult otherwise to explain the increased stature of people of many nations.

This is not to say that we now have the best diet possible. Most of us in the U.S. and in many other countries eat too much. The ideal amounts of animal fats, vegetable fats, proteins, carbohydrates, roughage, vitamins and minerals in the diet are still matters for investigation and debate. Even with our limited knowl-

MEDICINAL PLANTS on the opposite page are from a plate in *Culpeper's English Physician and Complete Herbal*, revised by E. Silby about 1798 and reproduced here through the courtesy of the Burndy Library. Written by Nicholas Culpeper (1616–1654), an English physician and astrologer, the book listed hundreds of plants that could be "applied to the cure of all disorders incident to mankind." For example, the inner bark from the elder (*top left*) "boiled in water, and drunk, purgeth exceedingly; berries green or dry often given with good success for the dropsy." Fennel was recommended to "break wind, provoke urine and ease the pains of, as well as break, the stone. The leaves, or rather seed, boiled in water, will stay the hiccough." Fern roots boiled in mead kill "worms in the body." Fern leaves, when eaten, purge "the belly of choleric and waterish humours, but they also trouble the stomach; they also cause abortion." Most of the concoctions described by Culpeper no longer have a place in the pharmacopoeia. One plant, however, the foxglove, is still very much in the picture. In Culpeper's time it was used in a potion for "feebleness of the heart" and as an emetic. Today it is the source of digitalis, which strengthens the contractions of the heart muscle. When weakness of heart muscle has caused water retention, digitalis may act as a diuretic.

edge, however, physicians are able to prescribe special diets that are clearly beneficial for people with certain inborn errors of metabolism. For example, sprue is an illness that often causes diarrhea and malnutrition because of poor absorption of food in the small intestine. The inborn error in sprue has not yet been discovered, but it is known that patients with sprue are intolerant of gluten, a sticky protein found in wheat and some other foods. As long as gluten is consumed, patients subject to sprue suffer from the symptoms of the disease. The delicately fringed microscopic lining of the small intestine becomes peculiarly blunted and inefficient. Good health can almost always be restored simply by omitting gluten from the diet.

Lactose, the sugar found in milk, is not itself absorbed in the bloodstream. Its molecule is first cleaved in the small intestine into the smaller molecules of glucose and galactose, two sugars that can be readily absorbed. The cleavage

of lactose into glucose and galactose is accomplished by an enzyme called lactase. After infancy some people develop a deficiency of lactase. When a person with a lactase deficiency drinks a large amount of milk, diarrhea and various kinds of abdominal discomfort often ensue. The remedy is a diet that does not contain lactose. Intolerance for lactose is an inherited metabolic trait.

Sprue and lactase deficiency illustrate a small number of conditions in which a specific diet constitutes effective chemical intervention. In some other illnesses, probably also of genetic origin, certain diets can provide partial or occasional relief. For example, there is one kind of diabetes (characterized by the excretion of glucose into the urine) that appears in people who are too fat. This diabetes is greatly ameliorated by a diet low enough in calories to ensure an optimal weight.

A number of diets that are of no proved value at all are widely publicized and sold. For example, some diets are

said to be therapeutic for various mental illnesses, but there is no proof that this is so. Others are based, mistakenly but profitably, on the notion that low blood sugar (hypoglycemia) is a very common ailment and aim to correct it even when it is not present. There are individuals who do show various types of periodic lowering of the blood-sugar concentration, but these illnesses are not common and should be diagnosed and treated only by a physician. In fact, if any unusual diet is embarked on, it should only be on a physician's advice.

The ready availability of pure vitamins has made it possible to halt many diseases that are caused by the absence of certain vitamins in the diet or by the inability to absorb them. Pernicious anemia, which was once invariably fatal, can now be managed with infrequent and inexpensive injections of vitamin B-12. Vitamins are often taken unnecessarily. Vitamin C prevents or cures scurvy, once a lethal disease of sailors and others long-removed from fresh fruits and vegetables, but there is no convincing evidence that it cures or prevents colds. Fortunately it is harmless, even in large doses, as are the B vitamins. Vitamins A and D, on the other hand, are poisonous in very large doses [*see illustration on opposite page*].

With some exceptions, tampering with ordinary nutritional habits is not beneficial. Nearly everyone with an adequate diet thrives, in spite of wide variations in what normal people eat. This is in striking contrast to the difficulties that may be encountered when, because of illness or accident or surgery, a patient cannot eat and must be nourished intravenously. Depending on the conditions, the problem may be relatively simple. For example, a patient who is otherwise well nourished and healthy but who cannot eat for a few days after surgery may require only appropriately sterile and optimal concentrations of glucose and salt.

The situation is quite different when the patient has extensive bowel disease and must be nourished intravenously for two months. A host of problems, some of them well understood and others poorly, confront the physician. He must worry about the concentration of such elements as sodium, potassium, calcium, magnesium and phosphorus. He must devise ways of infusing adequate amounts of protein or of amino acids, the molecules of which protein is made. Intravenous protein is expensive and carries with it some risks. Constant infusions require exceedingly careful techniques to avoid inflammation of the veins and serious

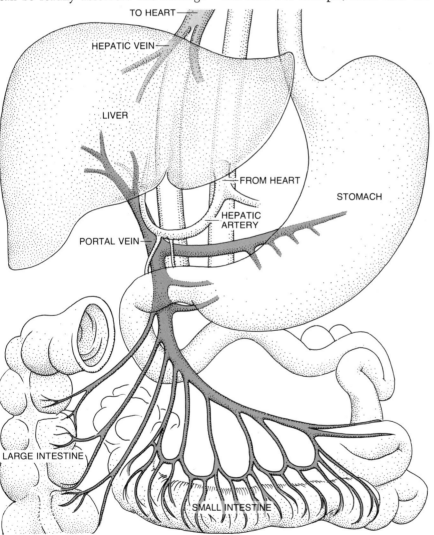

THE LIVER plays a key role in detoxifying ingested substances after they leave the stomach and intestines and before they reach the rest of the body. Many drugs taken to combat disease are destroyed by the liver because their chemical structure is similar to that of naturally occurring toxic substances. The liver also converts nutrients absorbed from the digestive tract into forms that are easier for the rest of the body to tolerate and utilize.

COMMON NAME	SOME CONDITIONS CAUSED BY DEFICIENCY	EFFECT OF EXCESS INGESTION
Vitamin A	Night blindness, some kinds of skin disease, poor fetal development	Mental disturbances, nausea, vomiting, skin and bone deformities
Vitamin B-1 (Thiamine)	Impairment of brain, nerves and heart	None
Vitamin B-2 (Riboflavin)	Poor function of nervous system	None
Niacin	Pellagra (diarrhea, inflamed skin, mental deterioration)	None, unless taken in the form of nicotinic acid
B-6 (Pyridoxine)	Poor function of nervous system, sometimes convulsions	None
B-12 (Cyanocobalamin)	Pernicious anemia (fatal failure in production of red blood cells and platelets, brain and nerve damage)	None
Vitamin C (Ascorbic acid)	Scurvy (swollen, bleeding gums and joints, mental disturbances)	None
Vitamin D	Poor absorption of calcium, poor development or maintenance of bones, irritability of nervous system	Abnormally high blood calcium, depression of brain function, kidney damage
Folic acid	Poor growth and development, anemia	None except that folic acid ingestion may mask pernicious anemia
Biotin	Some skin diseases	None
Pantothenic acid	Some nutritional disorders	None
Vitamin E	Poor red-cell survival in some infants	None
Vitamin K	Abnormal bleeding	None

VITAMINS REQUIRED BY MAN are listed, along with some of the conditions caused by the absence of vitamins and the effect of their excessive intake. The ideal amount of each vitamin (and most of the other essential foodstuffs) in the diet is not yet known.

infections. In spite of such difficulties chemical intervention to provide complete nutrition by intravenous feeding has been accomplished and is a monumental achievement.

The defenses of the body against invasion by bacteria, viruses and other microorganisms are numerous, complex and still not fully understood. Edward Jenner, an astute English physician, inaugurated vaccination against smallpox in 1796. In the 1880's Louis Pasteur devised a way of modifying the rabies virus to make possible immunization against that dreadful and nearly always fatal disease. In both cases the concept is similar: an agent that does not cause a serious illness is injected in order to stimulate the immune system of the body. The same principle now allows very effective immunization against poliomyelitis, tetanus, diphtheria and both kinds of measles (rubella and rubeola) [*see illustration on next page*].

Truly effective immunization not only prevents suffering, disability and death but also confers enormous economic benefits. For example, it has been estimated that the savings from poliomyelitis im-

munization in the U.S. alone (hospital costs, disability losses and so on) amount to between $100 million and $180 million per year. Savings of a similar magnitude have resulted from immunization against measles.

It is also sometimes possible to artificially provide missing elements of the natural defense system. For example, some people lack gamma globulin, the protein fraction of the blood that normally plays a critical role in defense against most infections. To protect such individuals gamma globulin can be given by injection. In rare circumstances transplantation of normal bone marrow, which manufactures the lymphocytes that produce antibodies, can be accomplished to restore normal immunity. There is much active research in the field of bone-marrow transplants. Another substance manufactured by the body in response to virus infections, interferon, tends to inhibit the spread of viruses. Various means of stimulating the body to produce interferon are being studied experimentally.

Many drugs have been developed that

suppress rather than assist the body's natural defenses against infection. Some of these drugs have value when, for reasons that are poorly understood, the body overreacts to a virus or to some other substance and produces antibodies or other destructive agents against itself. Common examples are severe asthma in reaction to plant pollen or to a virus or exaggerated blistering on exposure to poison oak. Much less common examples are diseases of unknown origin in which the immune defense mechanisms are so overactive as to be self-destructive. One of these diseases, Wegener's granulomatosis, may cause fatal ulceration of the air passages. Judicious use of drugs that suppress immune responses can bring the overreaction under control.

In organ-transplant operations the immune system of the recipient must be suppressed (unless the donor is an identical twin). Here again the physician must steer between Scylla and Charybdis. Too little immune suppression and the transplanted organ will be killed by antibodies. Too much immune suppression and bacteria or other invaders will kill the patient. Some drugs that are used to suppress the immune system, and others that interfere with the normal use of essential nutrients (antimetabolites), are helpful in suppressing certain forms of cancer, particularly those, such as leukemia, that involve the uncontrolled growth of white blood cells.

Hormones are the chemical messengers that regulate body functions. They are secreted by glands and by individual cells. Several of them are manufactured in the brain and other parts of the nervous system. The hormones play a major role in such diverse processes as growth, sexual development, emotions, the tempo of metabolism, the regulation of body temperature, the contraction of the heart, the combustion and storage of

sugar and fats, the conversion of protein to sugar and the elimination of wastes through the kidneys. Many diseases are caused by a deficiency or an excess of one hormone or more. For example, absence of insulin (one of the hormones secreted by cells in the pancreas) produces a kind of diabetes with very high blood sugar that is fatal unless insulin injections are given. On the other hand, too much insulin may be secreted by a tumor of the pancreas, and the oversupply of the hormone may cause intermittent loss of consciousness because of the deficiency of sugar in the blood.

There are now satisfactory remedies for most of the large number of illnesses caused by hormonal deficiency or excess.

Improved methods of treatment and diagnosis are becoming available. Recently the precise chemical structure of some hormones (including insulin) has been determined, and new methods of synthesizing hormones have been developed. No longer does the physician have to rely on crude hormonal extracts.

Some hormones are useful not only for making up hormonal deficiencies but also for treating a variety of illnesses that respond to an excess of a particular hormone. For example, some of the adrenocortical hormones can be administered to combat an exceedingly severe asthmatic constriction of the airways in the lungs. Noradrenalin, which increases the force of the heart contraction, is used to prevent death from very low blood pressure caused by acute serious injury.

DISEASE	CAUSATIVE AGENT	TYPE OF VACCINE	DURATION OF PROTECTION
Adenovirus infection	Virus	Killed Live	Short-lived Long-lasting
Bubonic plague	Bacterium	Killed Live	About six months About six months
Cholera	Bacterium	Killed	About six months
Diphtheria	Bacterium	Toxoid Antitoxin	Long-lasting Short-lived
German measles	Virus	Live	Long-lasting
Influenza	Virus	Killed	Short-lived
Measles	Virus	Live	Long-lasting
Mumps	Virus	Live	Long-lasting
Poliomyelitis	Virus	Live Killed	Long-lasting Two to four years
Rabies	Virus	Live Killed	Short-lived Short-lived
Rocky Mountain spotted fever	Rickettsia	Killed	Long-lasting
Smallpox	Virus	Live	Several years
Tetanus	Bacterium	Toxoid Antitoxin	Long-lasting Short-lived
Tuberculosis	Bacterium	Live	Long-lasting
Tularemia	Bacterium	Killed	Short-lived
Typhoid fever	Bacterium	Killed	Short-lived
Typhus	Rickettsia	Killed	About one year
Whooping cough	Bacterium	Killed	Probably permanent
Yellow fever	Virus	Live	About 10 years

PROTECTIVE IMMUNIZATION against the 19 diseases listed here is possible. All these measures have come in the 20th century except two: the smallpox vaccine (introduced by Edward Jenner in 1796) and the rabies vaccine (developed by Louis Pasteur in the 1880's).

The most widely used hormone prescription in the world today is "the pill." It consists of a combination of estrogens and progesterones that act to suppress ovulation. Chemically similar drugs are also used for birth control and in some cases for treating sterility in women. In general this form of chemical intervention has been very successful. The perfect solution to such problems has not yet been found, however. Apparently because of an inherited susceptibility to certain actions of the female hormones, some women who have taken the pill for a prolonged time develop liver impairment or high blood pressure.

In 1907 Paul Ehrlich of Germany, after long travail, succeeded in synthesizing Salvarsan, an arsenic compound that would kill *Treponema pallidum,* the microorganism that causes syphilis. Like many before him, Ehrlich was actually seeking a way to exterminate all disease-causing organisms in the body with one grand chemical blow. His dream is still not realized, but chemotherapy, the use of chemicals to control infections, is an enormously (not completely) successful chapter in the history of medicine. Sulfonamides, which are still useful in selected infections, were developed in the 1930's and 1940's. Alexander Fleming's discovery of penicillin and its development in the 1940's provided for the first time a drug with the power to kill bacteria in doses virtually harmless to man (apart from an occasional allergic reaction to the drug). Fleming's discovery and the subsequent work on penicillin by Howard Florey and Ernst Boris Chain generated a great and productive interest in antibiotics. Many diseases that were once fatal, for example bacterial infection of the heart valves, can now be cured. Many kinds of pneumonia

HORMONE	PRINCIPAL EFFECTS	SECRETED BY
Adrenocorticotropic hormone (ACTH)	Stimulates the adrenal cortex	Pituitary
Thyrotropin (TSH)	Stimulates the thyroid gland	Pituitary
Follicle-stimulating hormone (FSH)	Stimulates production of egg cells by ovary and spermatozoa by testes	Pituitary
Luteinizing hormone (LH)	Helps maturation of egg-bearing follicles in ovary or stimulates production of testosterone (male hormone) in testes	Pituitary
Growth hormone	Governs normal growth and helps to regulate metabolism	Pituitary
Prolactin	Regulates breast development and milk production	Pituitary
Antidiuretichormone (ADH), or Vasopressin	Regulates absorption of water in the kidney	Neurohypophysis (part of the pituitary)
Oxytocin	Facilitates movement of sperm in Fallopian tube, stimulates uterine muscle in childbirth, stimulates secretion of milk by breasts	Neurohypophysis
Cortisol and similar hormones	Regulate metabolism of sugar, protein, fat, minerals and water	Adrenal cortex (outer layer of adrenal gland)
Aldosterone and desoxycorticosterone	Regulate excretion and retention of minerals, particularly sodium and potassium, by kidneys	Adrenal cortex
Thyroid hormones	Regulate rate of body's metabolism	Thyroid
Estradiol 17-B ("Estrogen")	Regulates development of feminine characteristics and the menstrual-ovulatory cycle	Ovaries
Progesterone	Works with estrogen to regulate ovulation cycle and pregnancy. Estrogen-progesterone combinations, or similar agents, are the basis of birth-control pills	Ovaries
Testosterone	Regulates development of male characteristics and reproductive system	Testes
Insulin	Regulates utilization of sugar, proteins and fats	Pancreas (Islets of Langerhans)
Glucagon	Helps to regulate utilization of sugar, antagonizes insulin	Pancreas (Islets of Langerhans)
Parathyroid hormone	Regulates calcium metabolism	Parathyroid glands
Thyrocalcitonin	Helps to regulate calcium metabolism	Thyroid
Adrenalin	Stimulates brain and heart rate, mobilizes sugar and fat	Adrenal medulla (inner layer of adrenal gland)
Noradrenalin	Increases force of heart contraction and constricts arterioles	Adrenal medulla
Releasing factors	Individual ones cause release of ACTH, TSH, LH, FSH, prolactin and growth hormone by pituitary	Brain (hypothalamus)
Secretin	Stimulates pancreas to secrete chemicals needed for digestion of food	Lining of part of intestine
Cholecystokinin	Stimulates liver and pancreas to secrete chemicals needed in digestion, causes gall bladder to empty	Lining of part of intestine
Gastrin	Stimulates stomach to secrete hydrochloric acid	Lining of part of stomach and intestine

MAJOR HORMONES and the glands that secrete them are listed. Hormones are the chemical messengers that regulate body functions. They play a role in the metabolism of sugars, fats and proteins, and in growth, sexual development and blood circulation.

and infections of the lungs that were at best long and grave illnesses can now be cured easily and quickly if treated properly with antibiotics.

With the large assortment of antibiotics now available the physician must apply skill and wisdom in selecting the right one or the right combination. The selection depends on accurate diagnosis of the infection, consideration of the toxicity of the drug and the special characteristics of both the illness and the patient. A major problem with antibiotics, as with all useful drugs, is their injudicious use. No drug is a substitute for good sense. For example, it would be foolish to give chloramphenicol, a drug that can be lifesaving in typhoid fever but that occasionally destroys the bone marrow, to a patient with ordinary influenza. There are more subtle variations. Some doses of penicillin given before the offending bacteria are identified may render the exact diagnosis difficult or impossible to make. The aphorism "First give penicillin; if the patient does not recover, then examine him" is, alas, not always a joke.

CLASS	DRUG	PRESCRIBED FOR
Sulfonamides Sulfisoxazole		Infections of the urinary bladder
Penicillins Penicillin-G		Infections due to pneumococcus, streptococcus, gonococcus and meningococcus, and syphilis
Ampicillin Carbenicillin Oxacillin		Infections susceptible to penicillin and also some infections resistant to penicillin-G, for example penicillin-resistant staphylococci or bacilli that inhabit the bowel
Cephalosporins	Cephaloxin (oral) Cephalothin (injected)	Infections caused by bacilli in the bowel or on the skin
Aminoglycosides	Streptomycin	Tuberculosis, plague, tularemia
	Gentamicin	Severe infections caused by bacteria in the bowel
Polyenes	Amphotericin-B	Some fungus diseases, for example coccidioidomycosis and histoplasmosis
Tetracyclines	Tetracycline	Typhus, Rocky Mountain spotted fever, chancroid, granuloma inguinale, relapsing fever, psittacosis, lymphogranuloma venereum, atypical pneumonia, undulant fever
Lincomycins	Clindamycin	Infections caused by bacilli in the bowel
Miscellaneous	Chloramphenicol	Typhoid fever
	Isoniazid, ethambutol, rifampicin, cycloserine	Tuberculosis and similar infections
	Sulfones	Leprosy
	Piperazine citrate	Roundworm infestations
	Bephenium	Hookworm
	Thiabendazole	Roundworm infestations
	Niclosamide	Tapeworms
	Chloroquine	Some forms of malaria, amoeba or fluke infestations
	Diiodohydroxyquin	Amoeba infections
	Emetine	Amoeba infections
	Metronidazole	Amoeba and trichomonas infestations
	Quinine	Some forms of malaria
	Prionaquine	Some forms of malaria, trypanosomiasis (sleeping sickness)

ANTIMICROBIAL DRUGS now control many infections that were once leading causes of death. Sulfonamides were developed in the 1930's, penicillin in the 1940's. The best use of such drugs calls for accurate diagnosis and consideration of the drug's potential toxicity.

Periodically a new pain-relieving drug is announced with the claim that it is nonaddicting. So far no drug significantly more effective than aspirin in relieving real pain (as distinguished from anxiety or *Weltschmerz*) has been found that is not addicting to some extent, particularly if it is misused. Amphetamines that are prescribed for weight reduction or for depression also have some addiction potential and should be administered rarely and with much caution.

There are dozens of non-narcotic agents that affect mood or induce sleep, and none of them should be taken without the advice of a physician. In some circumstances such drugs are helpful in weathering minor emotional squalls, and some are used to treat major disorders such as schizophrenia. One recent discovery deserves special mention because of its specificity. It is lithium chloride, a naturally occurring salt that tastes like ordinary table salt. At one time lithium chloride was used as a salt substitute by individuals with high blood pressure or heart failure. When taken in large doses, it causes mental and nervous impairment, but in carefully regulated small doses it has no discernible effect in mentally normal people. When patients with manic-depressive psychosis are treated with lithium, however, their extreme mood swings are brought under control [see "Psychiatric Intervention," by Leon Eisenberg, page 79].

Parkinson's disease also produces changes in mood as well as physical impairment of the muscles and involuntary tremor. Pathologists had long noted that a part of the brain called the substantia nigra because of its black color was curiously blanched in people with Parkinson's disease. All black pigment (melanin) in the body is manufactured from the amino acid tyrosine, which is structurally related to substances known to affect the transmission of impulses between nerve cells. From these clues George C. Cotzias of the Brookhaven National Laboratory developed a way of treating Parkinson's disease with a chemical called levodopa, which is derived from tyrosine. Epilepsy is another illness of the nervous system that usually responds to chemical treatment. Dilantin, phenobarbital and a variety of newer drugs are available for the purpose. These drugs tend to depress some focus in the brain that is periodically overly excitable and causes seizures.

The circulation of the blood is beautifully adjusted to changes in the position of the body, to the level of physical exercise and to all the vicissitudes of man's life and the earth's variable environment. A wide variety of drugs that affect the circulation of the blood are available. The contractions of the heart muscle itself can be affected by digitalis, which has a strengthening effect in some kinds of heart failure but not in the normal heart. If part of the heart muscle is too irritable (as it sometimes is when its blood supply is inadequate), the focus of irritation may cause the heart to beat irregularly or too fast and result in inefficient pumping. Quinidine (derived from quinine) and other drugs that depress the irritability of the heart muscle can be prescribed to restore the normal rhythm and speed of the heart.

If the production of red blood cells in the bone marrow is inadequate, the result is anemia; if it is too exuberant, the result is polycythemia. Both can be treated successfully with drugs. The circulation of the blood can also be adversely affected when the kidneys do not excrete enough salt and water. The result is too high a blood volume. Many powerful drugs are now available for treating this condition.

The peripheral blood vessels can become overly constricted and cause high

CLASS	DRUG	PRESCRIBED FOR	ADVERSE REACTIONS
General anesthetics	Diethyl ether	General anesthesia (inhalation)	Explosion
	Nitrous oxide ("laughing gas")	General anesthesia (inhalation)	
	Halothane	General anesthesia (inhalation)	Liver damage
	Thiopental	General anesthesia (intravenous)	
Sedatives and hypnotics	Chloral hydrate	Insomnia	May be habit-forming
	Phenobarbital (long-acting)	Sedation, epilepsy	May be habit-forming
	Diazepam	Anxiety, insomnia	May be habit-forming
Anticonvulsants	Diphenylhydantoin	Epilepsy (grand mal)	Psychic disturbances, oversensitivity of gums
	Ethosuximide	Epilepsy (petit mal)	Disturbances of blood
Amine precursor	Levodopa	Parkinson's disease	Involuntary movements, Psychic changes
Analgesics	Acetylsalicylic acid (aspirin)	Pain, fever, inflammation	Bleeding from stomach
	Paracetamol	Pain, fever	Damage to red blood cells
Narcotic analgesics	Morphine	Severe pain	Depression of respiration, addiction
	Meperidine	Severe pain	Depression of respiration, addiction
	Codeine	Moderate pain, cough	Depression of respiration, addiction
	Methadone	Heroin addiction	Depression of respiration, addiction
Narcotic antagonists	Nalorphine	Narcotic analgesic overdosage	
Stimulants	Amphetamine	Appetite suppression, treatment of fatigue	Habit-forming
	Caffeine	Relief of fatigue	
Acetylcholine antagonists	Pilocarpine	Glaucoma	
	Atropine	Peptic ulcer	Acute glaucoma
	Succinylcholine	Muscle relaxation during anesthesia	Prolonged muscular paralysis
	Edrophonium	Myasthenia gravis	Slowing of heart
Norepinephrine antagonists	Ephedrine	Asthma	Rapid pulse
	Propranolol	Disorders of rhythm of heart	Heart failure, acute asthma
	Aldomet	High blood pressure	Liver damage, anemia, mental depression

DRUGS AFFECTING THE NERVOUS SYSTEM are useful in controlling a wide variety of ills, including pain, insomnia, fatigue, tremor, convulsions and mood disorders. Many drugs act on both the central nervous system and the autonomic nervous system. Drugs that are antagonists of acetylcholine or of norepinephrine, however, tend to act primarily on the autonomic nervous system.

blood pressure. In cases of shock the blood pressure falls drastically. In recent years many new drugs that dilate or compress the peripheral blood vessels have been developed.

The clotting of blood is a magnificently orchestrated process. Occasionally it fails because of some inborn error, as in hemophilia, or because one of the elements essential to clotting is missing, as when a virus drastically reduces the number of platelets (the tiny particles in the blood that initiate clotting) or when certain individuals have an exaggerated sensitivity to some drug that tends to prevent clotting (aspirin, for example). The clotting process may also go awry in the opposite direction. A clot, or thrombosis, may form inside a blood vessel and cut off the blood supply to some part of the body. We are all aware of the high toll when the thrombosis occurs in one of the arteries supplying the heart muscle (coronary occlusion) or the brain (stroke). Both bleeding and thrombosis can often be controlled by drugs or by injection of certain concentrated blood components.

From even a cursory review of the present means of intervening in the chemistry of the body several salient impressions emerge. The body chemistry is exceedingly complex and usually does not call for intervention. If it does require intervention, the less the better. No drug, however helpful, is totally lacking in risk for the person who receives it. Since chemical intervention is a two-edged sword, there is not much to protect the individual patient except the experience and judgment of his physician. Guardians of public health, such as the Food and Drug Administration, can under the best conditions pass on the general value of any specific drug. A chemical that can save the life of one patient, however, may hasten the death of another. Cortisone helps to sustain good health in patients who would otherwise die from destruction of the adrenal glands (Addison's disease), but Addison's disease can be confused with many other illnesses that are made worse by cortisone. In fact, more cortisone than the individual needs can cause serious illness. Some drugs are well tolerated by the large majority of people but cause grave illness in the few who have an inborn susceptibility to the substance. Thus when regulatory agencies approve a drug, they make possible use, abuse and misuse. It is impossible to have foolproof safeguards. If such agencies regulate too stringently, they are likely to cripple medical progress.

VIII

Psychiatric Intervention

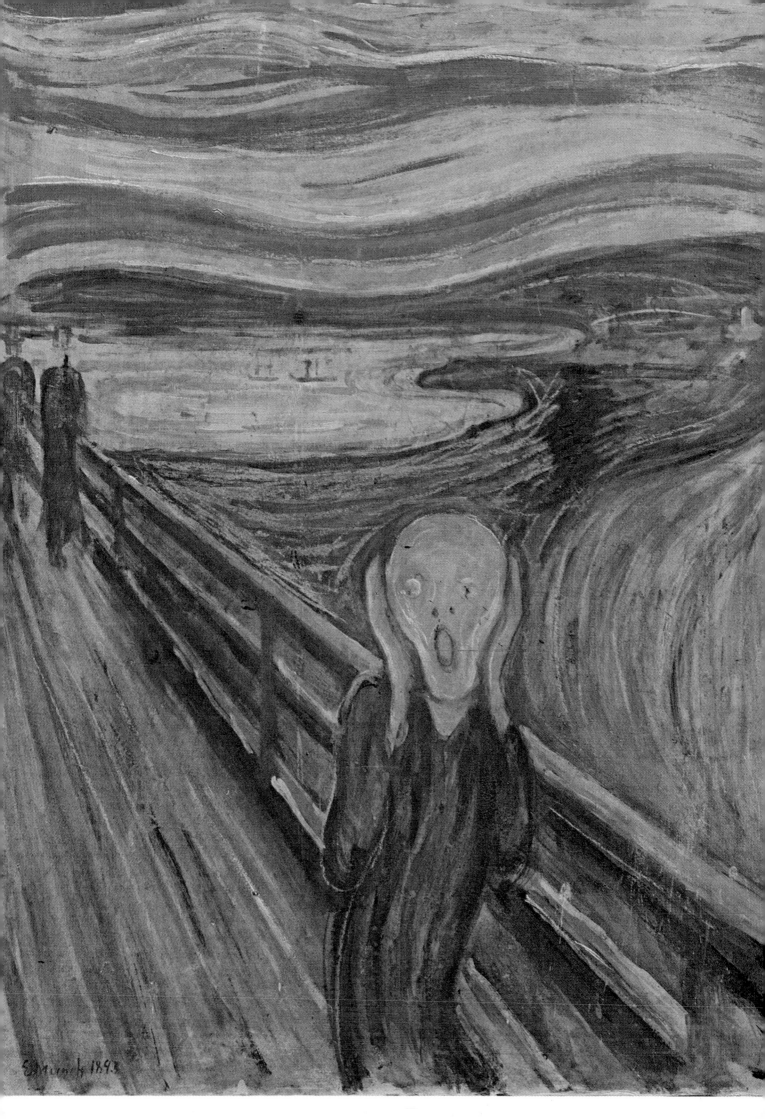
E Munch 1893

Psychiatric Intervention

LEON EISENBERG

Although enduring remedies for mental disorders are elusive, psychoactive drugs and community treatment programs have markedly reduced the number of people in mental hospitals

The course and outcome of the major mental disorders of man have been profoundly altered by the advent of drug treatment and by changes in the methods of delivering health care. These gains have been made in spite of our continuing ignorance of the basic causes and mechanisms of mental disorders. The remarkable efficacy of chemotherapy has provided a major spur to basic research into the biochemical and genetic mechanisms underlying psychiatric illness, and recent discoveries hold great promise for new and better means of diminishing the misery associated with disorders of the mind. The potential power of this developing "psychotechnology" is, however, creating concern about unwarranted intrusions into personal privacy and individual rights.

Even though large gains have been made, there remain major areas that await the impetus of new ideas and better methods. Psychotherapy (the psychological treatment of mental disorders) has many sources, but in the U.S. it took root in the soil provided by psychoanalysis. Whatever its future evolution, dynamic psychotherapy has had a powerful humanizing influence on medicine. It requires the physician to listen and to try to understand the patient rather than merely to categorize his foibles while remaining indifferent to his suffering.

The majority of patients with neuroses (disorders characterized by anxiety or psychic defenses that seek to ward off anxiety) describe themselves as being improved after psychotherapy. The symptomatic changes, however, appear to be nonspecific. Similar rates of improvement are found following treatments based on theories in complete contradiction to one another, and sometimes following the mere anticipation of treatment.

Psychoanalysis has undergone many changes since Freud's original formulations. Its theories, however, rest on argument, in the philosophical sense, rather than on evidence that meets the canons of science. Behavior therapy (based on conditioning theory) has shaken psychiatric traditionalism. Its usefulness for particular symptoms such as phobias would now be acknowledged by most psychiatrists, but its more general applicability remains to be demonstrated. Family-therapy methods have administered another jolt to conventional psychiatric thought. Its practitioners reformulate the problem from one "in" the patient to one "between" the patient and his family. The designated patient may merely be the scapegoat. The illness to be treated lies in distorted interpersonal relationships in the family. These concepts have broadened the psychiatrist's frame of reference. Family therapy, however, has spread more as a messianic movement and not because of convincing evidence from well-designed therapeutic trials.

Whether the psychological treatment of neurotic patients is an exclusive medical specialty is dubious. Such studies as we have provide no evidence that psychiatrists are more effective therapists than psychologists, social workers and counselors. Therefore in this article I concentrate on the major responsibility of psychiatry: the care and treatment of serious mental illness. It must be emphasized, however, that psychological judgment and personal sensitivity are indispensable to the effective function of the psychiatrist as a physician.

The severe mental disorders we have learned to deal with more effectively are the psychoses, the most prominent of which are schizophrenia and manic-depressive psychosis. Psychoses are severe disorders characterized by profound and pervasive alterations of mood, disorganization of thought and withdrawal from social interactions into fantasy. Schizophrenia is a psychosis with disturbances in the evaluation of reality and in conceptual thinking that are often accompanied by hallucinations and delusions. It usually becomes manifest in late adolescence or young adulthood. Manic-depressive psychosis is marked by severe disturbances in mood that are self-limited in time but are recurrent and frequently cyclic. Mania is manifested by psychic elation, increased motor activity, rapid speech and the quick flight of ideas. The stigmata of depression are melancholia, the slowing of thought, unusual thought content (for example overwhelming guilt over imagined transgressions and delusions of rotting away), motor retardation, sleep disturbances and preoccupation with bodily complaints.

The most obvious indicator of the ex-

"THE SCREAM" (*opposite page*), painted by Edvard Munch in 1893, captures the sensation of near-psychotic fear and despair. The original experience is described in Munch's diary: "I was walking along with two friends. Then the sun set...and melancholy overcame me. My friends went on, I stood alone, trembling with fright. I felt as if a great scream was going through nature." Psychiatrists have long been interested by the degree to which an artist's work reflects his personality, and Munch's works have been a popular subject of such studies. After completing the painting, Munch himself wrote: "Only someone insane could paint this!" The painting now hangs in the National Gallery in Oslo.

tent of the recent change in psychiatric practices is evident in the number of resident patients in the state and county mental hospitals of the U.S. [see illustration on page 82]. The number of patients peaked at about 560,000 in 1955. Over the preceding decade the number of patients had increased at the rate of 3 percent per year, almost twice the rate of growth of the population. Then the trend reversed sharply. The resident state and county mental-hospital population fell to 276,000 by 1972, in spite of general population growth and increased rates for both first admissions and readmissions. From 1962 to 1969 first-admission rates rose from 130,000 to 164,000 and readmission rates from 150,000 to 216,000 as the number of resident patients fell from 516,000 to 370,000. These figures reflect the dramatic decline in the average length of stay.

Although these data convey an overall picture of national trends, they fail to portray the extent of change in some areas. At present California has only some 5,400 patients in its state hospitals, a reduction of 80 percent since 1961, and it plans to eliminate all state-hospital beds for mental patients by 1977. Lest this be mistaken for the elimination of mental illness in California, or even the elimination of inpatient care as a mode of treatment, it should be noted that the state plan projects the transfer of care of mental patients to the counties. California counties now operate, in more or less adequate fashion, programs for the mentally ill, including psychiatric inpatient units in general hospitals and beds in nursing homes.

The total number of patient-care episodes (inpatient plus outpatient) in the U.S. increased from 1,675,000 in 1955 to 4,038,000 in 1971. In that period the number of inpatient episodes rose from 1,296,000 to 1,721,000, and the number of outpatient episodes zoomed from 379,000 to 2,317,000. Placed in relation to population growth, inpatient episodes per 100,000 population rose marginally from 799 to 847, whereas outpatient episodes increased from 234 to 1,134. The locus of care has shifted from the isolated and neglected wards of

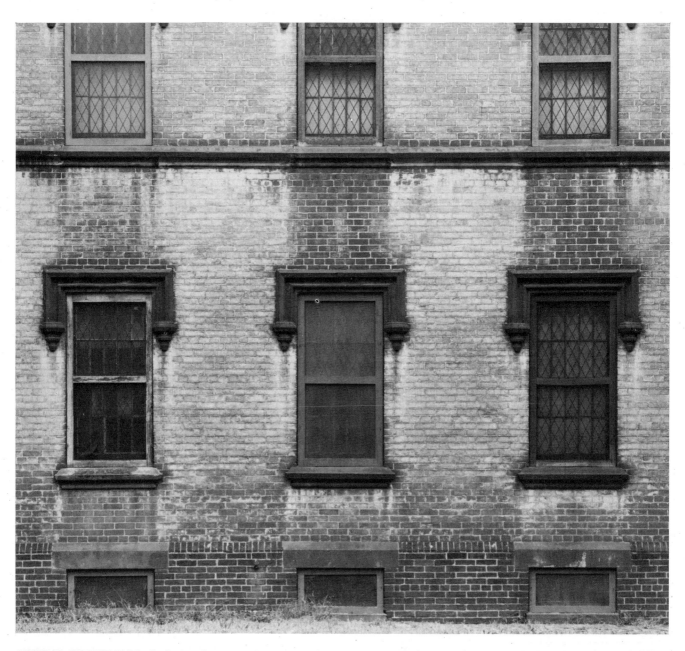

MENTAL HOSPITALS built during the past 100 years initially were an enlightened attempt to provide professional, institutionalized treatment for the mentally ill. Insufficient funding and public neglect, however, turned many of these hospitals into prison-like institutions, with badly deteriorated facilities. This building at St. Elizabeth's Hospital in Washington is no longer in use.

the state hospital to newly created but not always adequate facilities in the community. There is growing evidence that some of the former hospital patients are not cared for by anyone; they live in single-room-occupancy units, kinless and friendless, subsisting marginally on welfare allotments. Given what most state mental hospitals once were and what many still are, most patients are better off out of them than in them. This, however, does not excuse our failure to provide for the patients lost in the shuffle from one pattern of care to another.

The net change in patient treatment has been enormous, with the number of patients in state and county mental hospitals reduced by half, with the great majority of patients spending less time in the hospital for a given episode of illness and with far fewer of those admitted being condemned to an endless hospital stay. What factors account for these dramatic changes? Although a complete explanation is lacking, two important transformations in psychiatric care have played the major roles. They are the rediscovery of the principles of moral (that is, humane) treatment and the development of effective psychotropic drugs.

Responding to the humanistic ideas of the revolutionary era of the 18th century, Vincenzo Chiarugi of Italy, Philippe Pinel of France and William Tuke of England pioneered in the recognition that the way mental patients are treated affects the way they behave.

Chiarugi wrote into the regulations of the Bonifacio hospital in Florence in 1788 the statement: "It is a supreme moral duty and medical obligation to respect the insane person as an individual." The famous engraving of Pinel striking the chains from the insane at the Bicêtre (an accomplishment he modestly credited to his nonmedical hospital governor, Jean-Baptiste Pussin) symbolizes, if it also mythologizes, his accomplishment. In Pinel's words: "In lunatic hospitals, as in despotic governments, it is no doubt possible to maintain, by unlimited confinement and barbarous treatment, the appearance of order and loyalty. The stillness of the grave and the silence of death, however, are not to be expected in a residence consecrated for the re-

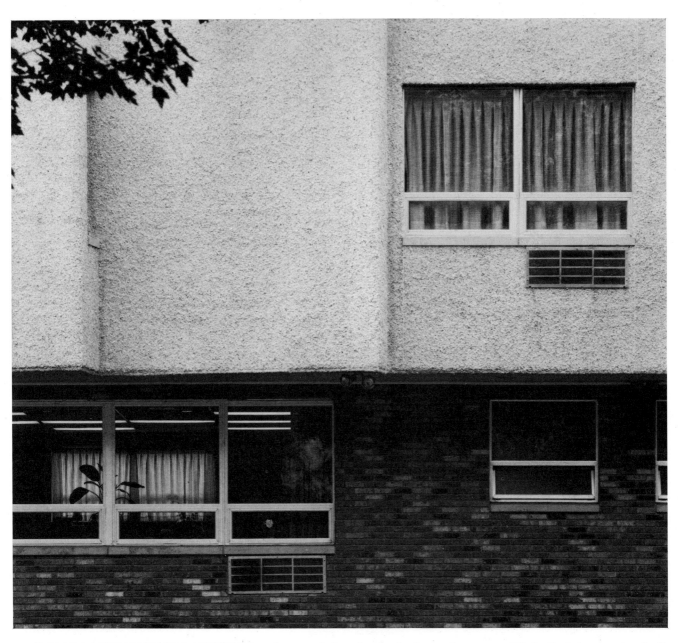

COMMUNITY MENTAL-HEALTH CENTERS have been established in the past few years throughout the U.S. with funding support from the National Institute of Mental Health. It is expected that in the future the centers will obtain their operating funds from state and local sources. Typical of the new community centers is the one at Dumont, N. J., where this photograph was taken.

---

ception of madmen. A degree of liberty, sufficient to maintain order, dictated not by weak but enlightened humanity and calculated to spread a few charms over the unhappy existence of maniacs, contributes in most instances to diminish the violence of symptoms and in some to remove the complaint altogether."

In England, Tuke and the Society of Friends founded The Retreat at York. They chose the name to suggest "a quiet haven in which the shattered bark might find the means of reparation or of safety." Samuel Tuke, grandson of the founder, wrote in a description of the moral treatment of the insane: "If it be true, that oppression makes a wise man mad, is it to be supposed that stripes, and insults, and injuries, for which the receiver knows no cause, are calculated to make a madman wise? Or would they not exasperate his disease, and excite his resentment?"

These quotations convey the extent to which convictions about the centrality of human liberty gave rise to a therapeutic philosophy that came to replace confinement and punishment. Succeeding waves of neglect, reform and neglect of institutional patient treatment led a century and a half later to state mental hospitals that were unmanageably large, poorly staffed and grossly underfunded. These self-contained worlds became dedicated to self-perpetuation rather than to the patients to whom they were ostensibly dedicated.

In the late 1940's and early 1950's there were two significant developments. First, sociologists began to examine the nature of mental institutions and the interactions of patients and staff as these influenced the behavior of the patient. Second, innovative hospital superintendents, first in Britain and then in the U.S., opened locked doors, introduced a measure of patient self-government and reestablished bonds with the surrounding community. It soon became evident that the apparently deteriorated behavior of chronic mental patients was not a simple result of the mental disorder that had led to admission but of what has been termed the social-breakdown syndrome, that is, the alienation and dehumanization produced by the "total institution" the mental hospital had become. With a reconceptualization of the hospital as a therapeutic community (the new name for moral treatment), many of the chronic inpatients were able to be returned to the community, even after years of continuous hospitalization, and far fewer first admissions became chronic.

The reversal of the continuous growth of the inpatient population began with the reordering of the institutional environment, the development of community-care alternatives, changes in administrative policy favoring early discharge, and hard-won battles for community acceptance of the mentally ill. Although the first decrease of the inpatient population preceded the large-scale introduction of drug treatment, the continued and much higher rate of change would not have been possible unless effective chemotherapeutic means of managing acute psychotic disorders had become available at the same time.

The history of psychopharmacology can readily be made to fit Horace Walpole's parable of the "Three Princes of Serendip," but it may be more instructive to recall Louis Pasteur's aphorism that chance favors the prepared mind. Chlorpromazine, the prime example of the new psychotherapeutic drugs, resulted from efforts to synthesize a more effective antihistamine. In 1949 Henri-Marie Laborit of France used chlorpromazine to produce a "hibernation syndrome" in patients undergoing prolonged surgery, and he noticed that a side effect was a striking indifference to environmental stimuli. Then in 1952 Jean Delay and Pierre Deniker of France discovered the drug's remarkable effectiveness in aborting acute psychotic episodes, both in schizophrenia and in the manic phase of manic-depressive disorders. The confirmation of chlorpromazine's quite extraordinary value by controlled clinical trials led to its widespread use throughout the world and to an organized search for related families of compounds, a search that required close interaction of organic chemists, pharmacologists and clinicians. New classes of drugs now termed major tranquilizers or neuroleptics were discovered.

In spite of the similarity of these drugs in pharmacologic properties, they vary in chemical structure, milligram-for-milligram potency, in frequency of side effects and in their utility for the treatment of clinical subtypes within the schizophrenic spectrum. (For example, trifluoperazine is thought to be more useful for the inhibited schizophrenic and chlorpromazine for the overactive schizophrenic.) Extensive clinical research has documented the effectiveness of the phenothiazine class of drugs (which includes chlorpromazine and trifluoperazine) in terminating an episode of schizophrenia. The natural history of the disorder, how-

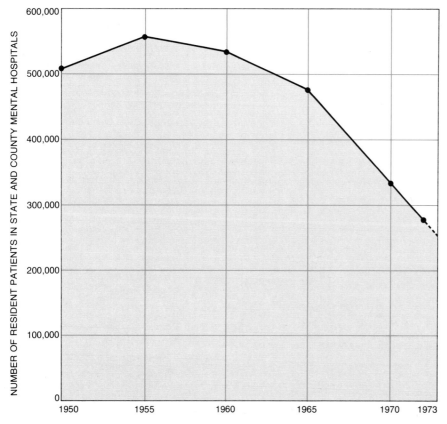

NUMBER OF RESIDENT PATIENTS at year-end in state and county mental hospitals is shown for the period 1950 to 1972. The resident mental-patient population peaked in 1955. The data were provided by the Biometry Branch of the National Institute of Mental Health.

ever, indicates a substantial risk of recurrence and little residue of benefit from prior treatment. Studies of maintenance therapy, when the patient is willing and able to take an appropriate drug over a long period of time, indicate a definite attenuation in the rate of subsequent attacks. Unfortunately unpleasant side effects (sedation and symptoms resembling Parkinson's disease) are a problem for some patients and serious toxicity (persistent rhythmical, involuntary movements of tongue and face, abnormal pigmentation, low white-cell count and jaundice) afflicts a substantial minority.

Ayurvedic medicine in India had for thousands of years made use of the snakeroot plant, *Rauwolfia serpentina*, for its sedative properties. When rauwolfia was introduced as an antihypertensive agent in the late 1940's and early 1950's, its active principle, reserpine, was identified. One serious side effect was the production of severe depression in some patients. The introduction of reserpine into psychiatry led to the discovery of the drug's effectiveness in aborting acute psychotic episodes in schizophrenia. Once widely used, reserpine has been replaced by the phenothiazines because of the greater frequency of reserpine's serious side effects. It continues, however, to play an important role in the experimental pharmacology of the psychoses.

In the same year that chlorpromazine was introduced into psychiatry alert clinicians treating tuberculosis with iproniazid noted that many of their patients displayed a marked euphoria well before there was any major improvement in their pulmonary disease. Subsequent trials in depressed patients established the power of this agent in relieving depression. It was also discovered that iproniazid acted to inhibit the enzyme monamine oxidase. (Monamines, such as serotonin, norepinephrine and dopamine, are believed to act as chemical transmitters between nerve cells in the brain.) At about the same time organic chemists synthesized the drug imipramine by replacing the sulfur atom in the phenothiazine structure with a dimethyl bridge, thereby changing a six-member ring into a seven-member ring. Tests with animals had suggested that imipramine should have properties similar to the parent compound, but the drug proved relatively ineffective in schizophrenics.

In 1957, however, R. Kuhn of Switzerland, observing that depressed schizophrenics did seem to show some im-

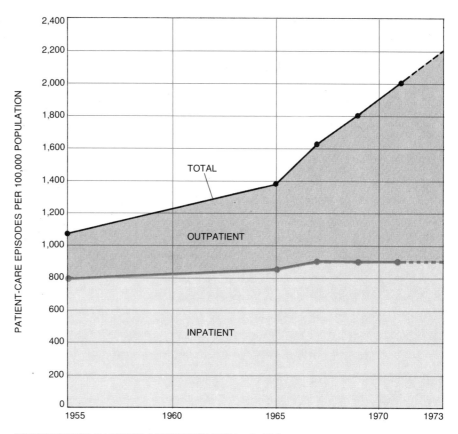

PSYCHIATRIC PATIENT-CARE EPISODES in the U.S. per 100,000 population are shown. The rate of outpatient care has doubled since 1965, and accounts for nearly all the increase in the total patient-care rate. The inpatient-care rate has held steady for more than a decade.

provement on being given imipramine, demonstrated that patients suffering from psychotic depression displayed marked improvement. Imipramine was the prototype of the tricyclic antidepressants. The chemical structures of these two classes of antidepressants—the monamine oxidase inhibitors and the tricyclics—are quite different [*see illustration on next page*]. The drugs are effective in the management of from 70 to 80 percent of depressive episodes and have much reduced the reliance on electroconvulsive therapy, which was once the only known effective treatment for depressive illness. In Australia J. F. J. Cade was pursuing the hypothesis that mania was the result of a toxic state that he sought to detect by searching for metabolic products in the urine. Having employed lithium because of the solubility of its urate salt, he noted that the lithium given to laboratory animals acted as a sedative. He then used it in clinical trials that indicated the element could control mania. Cade's lead was ignored for more than a decade because of concern about lithium toxicity, which had become disturbingly evident when its salts were imprudently administered in high doses as a substitute for sodium in the treatment of hypertension. With proper attention

to dosage and careful monitoring of levels in the blood serum, lithium has now been shown to be a safe agent for the treatment of mania, although it is not as prompt in its action as chlorpromazine. The most exciting development has been the demonstration by the Danish group headed by Mogens Schou that lithium is an effective prophylactic agent against the recurrence of psychotic episodes in patients with manic-depressive disease. For the first time we have an agent with acceptably low levels of toxicity (under close medical supervision), low cost and ease of administration that prevents to a significant degree the otherwise inevitable recurrent attacks of a major psychosis.

Studies of the biochemistry of the brain, which were stimulated in large part by the desire to understand how the psychoactive drugs worked, indicate that selective errors in the metabolism of the monamines in specific areas of the brain may be the pathophysiological basis for psychotic disorders. Chemical and histological studies indicate that these substances are located in certain nerve cells and the ends of their long fibers. The biogenic amines (including serotonin, norepinephrine and dopamine) most likely function in specific regions of the central nervous system as chemical transmitters between nerve cells or as modulators of transmission by other substances (such as acetylcholine).

There appears to be a close relation between the effects of the psychoactive drugs on monamine levels and on affective and behavioral states. Drugs that result in an inactivation and depletion of norepinephrine in the brain (such as reserpine and lithium) produce sedation and depression. Drugs such as imipramine, together with monamine oxidase inhibitors that increase or potentiate norepinephrine, are associated with behavioral stimulation and usually have an antidepressant effect in man. Therefore abnormally high or low levels of norepinephrine in functionally specialized areas of the brain may be responsible for at least some types of elation and depression.

There is growing evidence that the metabolic substance cyclic AMP mediates some of the effects of norepinephrine and dopamine in the brain. For example, in the brain structure called the caudate nucleus dopamine stimulates the activity of adenylate cyclase,

NAME	MOLECULAR STRUCTURE	PRESCRIBED FOR	TYPICAL DAILY ORAL DOSE
NEUROLEPTICS PHENOTHIAZINES	CHLORPROMAZINE TRIFLUOPERAZINE	SCHIZOPHRENIA, MANIA SCHIZOPHRENIA, MANIA	400 – 800 MILLIGRAMS 15 – 40 MILLIGRAMS
RAUWOLFIA	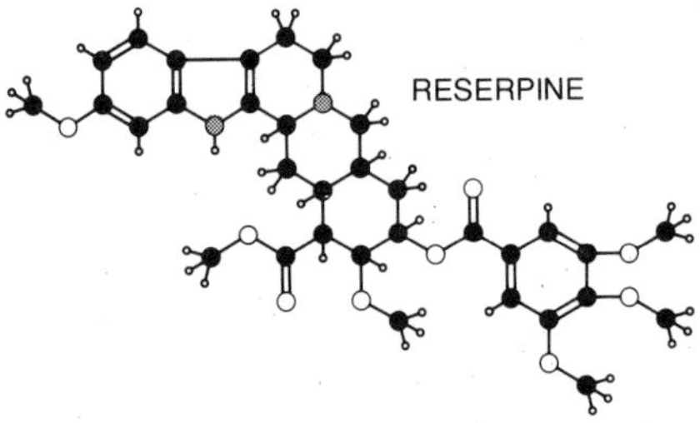 RESERPINE	SCHIZOPHRENIA, MANIA	4 – 10 MILLIGRAMS
ANTIDEPRESSANTS TRICYCLICS	IMIPRAMINE NORTRIPTYLINE	DEPRESSION DEPRESSION	100 – 300 MILLIGRAMS 20 – 100 MILLIGRAMS
MONAMINE OXIDASE INHIBITORS	NIALAMIDE PHENELZINE	DEPRESSION DEPRESSION	50 – 200 MILLIGRAMS 20 – 60 MILLIGRAMS
PROPHYLACTIC AGENT	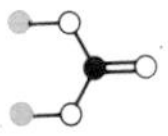 LITHIUM CARBONATE	MANIA, PREVENTION OF RECURRENCE OF MANIC-DEPRESSIVE DISORDERS	900 – 1,500 MILLIGRAMS

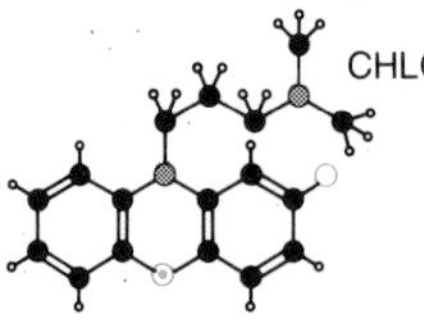

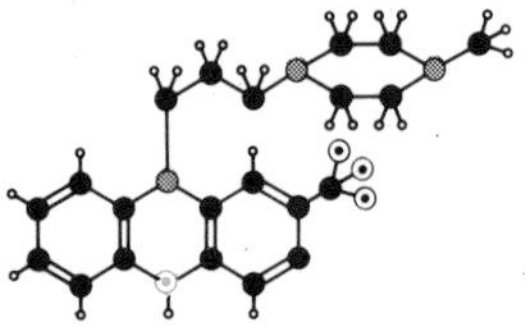

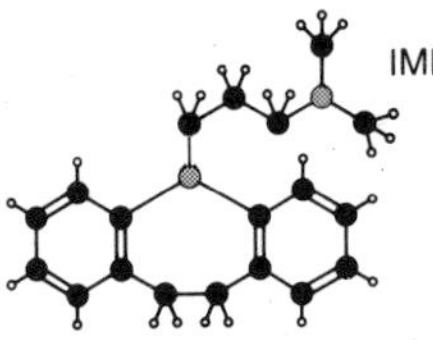

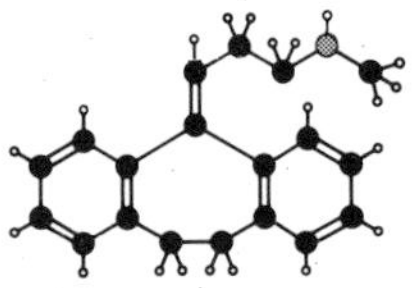

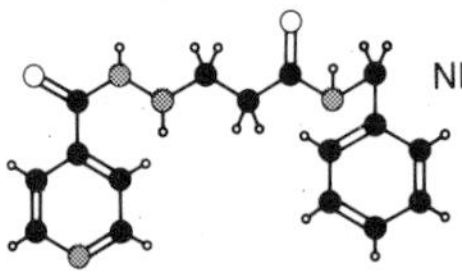

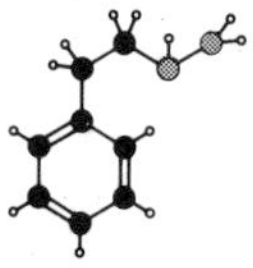

○ OXYGEN ● LITHIUM
● CARBON ○ CHLORINE
• HYDROGEN ⊙ FLUORINE
◉ NITROGEN ⊙ SULFUR

MAJOR CLASSES OF DRUGS prescribed for the treatment of schizophrenia or manic-depressive disorders are listed along with representative examples of each class. In addition the chemical

the enzyme that catalyzes the synthesis of cyclic AMP from adenosine triphosphate. Cyclic AMP is present in large concentrations in the central nervous system and is known to be important in the induction of enzymes and the synthesis of other proteins. Recent experiments have indicated that protein synthesis may play an important role in long-term memory. When chemicals that inhibit

SIDE EFFECTS
DROWSINESS, HYPOTENSION, EXTRAPYRAMIDAL SYMPTOMS (MASKLIKE FACE, RIGIDITY, TREMOR), WEIGHT INCREASE, ALLERGIC REACTIONS IN LIVER, SKIN AND BLOOD
NASAL STUFFINESS, NAUSEA, DIARRHEA, WORSENING OF PEPTIC ULCER, DEPRESSION
HYPOTENSION, DRY MOUTH, BLURRED VISION, URINARY RETENTION, DROWSINESS, INCREASED INTRAOCULAR PRESSURE
HYPOTENSION, DROWSINESS, HYPERTENSIVE CRISES AFTER INGESTION OF FOOD WITH TYRAMINE (SUCH AS AGED CHEESE)
TREMOR, NAUSEA, WEAKNESS, GASTRIC DISCOMFORT, GOITER

structure, typical range of dosage and primary side effects are given for each example.

protein synthesis are injected into the brain of an experimental animal, the formation of long-term memories is suppressed. Drugs that release or enhance norepinephrine in the brain counteract this suppression. These findings, made by Seymour S. Kety of the Harvard Medical School, support a tentative model of memory in which protein synthesis stimulated by the release of norepinephrine serves as the biochemical basis for the consolidation of learning. Although there are no completely adequate theories to account for the correlation between biochemical change, nerve-cell activity and behavior, the exciting pace of interchange between clinical studies and laboratory investigations promises major gains in our understanding of the fundamental mechanisms.

Evidence has been accumulating that points toward a genetic basis for schizophrenia and for manic-depressive disorders. The risk of schizophrenia for a child with one schizophrenic parent is about 10 times greater than it is in the general population, and the risk for a child with two schizophrenic parents is about 40 times greater. This empirical finding can be explained on either a genetic basis or an environmental one. Research on twins, however, has shown that schizophrenia in both twins is much commoner (with a range of 35 to 70 percent) in monozygotic (identical) pairs than it is (with a range of 10 to 26 percent) in dizygotic (fraternal) pairs.

A continuing American-Danish study conducted by Kety, D. Rosenthal, P. H. Wender and F. Schulsinger has provided independent evidence for a hereditary basis for schizophrenia. They have been studying people who as children were adopted and as adults became schizophrenic. A comparison of the prevalence of schizophrenia among the biological relatives of such people and among the adopting families makes it possible to separate the genetic component from the environmental one. The investigators have found more instances of schizophrenia and related disorders in biological relatives than in the adopting families, which offers strong support for genetic (although not Mendelian) transmission.

The emergence of these mental disorders probably requires a predisposition involving more than one gene (polygenic transmission) and still unspecified environmental precipitants. Studies of manic-depressive disorders in families indicate the need to differentiate bipolar disorders (with both manic and depressive episodes) from unipolar ones (with only depressive episodes). The prevalence of such disorders in the parents and extended family of bipolar patients is significantly greater than it is in the families of unipolar patients. The rates for families in both groups, however, are higher than they are for the general population.

Psychiatry, like the representation of the Roman god Janus, has two faces, one represented by treatment at the psychosocial level and the other by treatment at the pharmacologic level. The two forms of treatment often act to reinforce each other. Yet on the one hand the responsiveness of psychotic states to factors in the social environment has been taken to support contemporary views that mental illness is a "myth" arising from labels applied by psychiatrists in order to rationalize the segregation of people who exhibit disturbing (rather than disturbed) behavior. On the other, the power of psychotherapeutic drugs has been used to support a vulgarized medical model that views psychoses as nothing more than biochemical derangements to be corrected by a realignment of the biochemical machinery. Neither conclusion is warranted. The fundamental task of psychiatry is to understand behavior that results from interaction of stimulus (environmental) conditions and the response (psychobiological) capacities of the organism, capacities that reflect the organism's genetic endowment as well as its history (experience).

The notion that psychiatrists create insanity simply by labeling objectionable people as being insane has a certain charm. It implies that we can legislate mental illnesses out of existence by abolishing the myth that they are real. However, either this myth in one form or another has mysteriously proved to be necessary in every society or mental illnesses are in fact endemic in every population known to us. Studies of the lifetime expectancy for schizophrenia in Switzerland, Iceland and Japan reveal rates that vary only slightly: from .73 percent to 1.23 percent. The modal figure for all nations reporting is $1 \pm .2$ percent.

Some have argued that the frantic pace of industrialization increases psychotic behavior. H. Goldhammer and A. W. Marshall of the Rand Corporation compared the hospital rates for the psychoses of early and middle adult life in Massachusetts from 1840 to 1940. They found no substantial change.

The major psychoses are identifiable in preindustrial societies, although the local terms for them and the theories on which the terms are based differ sharply from our own. Both psychiatrists with Western training and native healers nonetheless identify a person with a psychosis as being abnormal. Mental disorders are identifiable even when the indigenous language has no verbal label for them and even when they are not defined as illness, as in senility. The signs and symptoms of mental deterioration are known to the community, but they are ascribed to the natural course of aging. The absence of the label does not abolish the behavior, but it does reflect a difference in social management; the patient's family, rather than some other community institution, assumes the burden of the affected person's care and protection.

Whatever the cause of a psychotic disorder, be it biological or psychogenic, the mental content of the psychosis must reflect the input to the mind and how that input is refracted by the mind's history and functional state. A patient

DOPAMINE

NOREPINEPHRINE

SEROTONIN

● CARBON   ○ OXYGEN
o HYDROGEN   ◐ NITROGEN

THREE CHEMICAL SUBSTANCES found at the ends of certain nerve fibers in the brain are depicted. The substances are thought to be involved in the transmission of signals between nerve cells. Drugs such as reserpine and lithium that deplete norepinephrine produce sedation and depression. Imipramine, which acts to potentiate norepinephrine, has an antidepressant effect.

suffering from a psychosis secondary to drug intoxication can only verbalize his hallucinations in the language he knows; he employs the images of his culture in expressing his terror. A schizophrenic with delusions of grandeur will think himself Jesus in one society and Mohammed in another. This does not say that the delusions were caused by the society but rather that the metaphors for grandeur are social in their origin. Moreover, if the psychotic abandons his insistence on being the deity in response to sympathy and support, that in itself does not tell us anything about the pathogenesis of the autistic thought.

Whether the patient is wildly delusional or rigidly catatonic, he remains a person in need of human satisfactions and he is always responsive to cues in his environment. Physicians quite regularly observe that the perceived pain of cancer, the visible tremor of neurological disease, the symptomatic malfunction of the lungs in emphysema increase or decrease in response to social transactions, which have awesome power to diminish or augment stress. The capacity of sedatives to diminish anxiety by damping physiological oscillations does not deny that the source of the anxiety lies in a psychological threat to personal esteem. The signs and symptoms of disordered function are a result of the state of the organism and the psychobiological forces acting on it.

The interactions among drug effects, psychobiological state and social setting indicate the complexity of the determinants of human behavior. Amphetamines, which for most of us are stimulants and euphoriants, are almost totally ineffective in the treatment of psychotic depression. Tricyclics, in spite of their potency in relieving depressed patients, produce nothing more than sedation and unpleasant side effects (dry mouth, blurring of vision and the like) in normal people. Lithium, which limits the swings of mood in manic-depressives, is without detectable effects in normal volunteers. An acutely psychotic patient may require for therapeutic benefit an amount of chlorpromazine capable of producing coma in a normal person. The perception of side effects, such as the dry mouth a patient has been warned to expect, may convince him of the potency and predictability of the drug and enhance favorable outcomes. For others a side effect such as sedation may arouse fears of losing self-control and result in refusal to continue treatment.

Social context affects a person's subjective response to drugs. Hallucinogens

evoke different experiences when they are given as a hallowed act in a religious ceremony, when they are part of a carefully monitored laboratory experiment or when they are taken in the search for "expanded consciousness." The effect depends on what the seeker expects and on whether he is alone or with others (the set and setting). Epinephrine (adrenaline) has been shown to produce irritation and anger when it is injected into a volunteer who does not know what he is receiving and is then exposed to a provocative and unpleasant situation. It generates feelings of well-being when it is injected into a person who is then exposed to a situation that is cheerful and humorous.

What transforms a troubled person into a patient (someone identified by himself, or his community, and a physician as being sick) is a complex social process influenced by cultural attitudes, medical knowledge and the availability of treatment facilities. It has long been observed that proximity to a state mental hospital, belief in the efficacy of psychiatric treatment and administrative policy facilitating easy access all lead to higher admission rates. Conversely, shame about mental illness, guilt about its cause and fear of long-term confinement are deterrents to acknowledging the need for help. Neither set of factors alters the actual prevalence of mental disorder, but they have a marked influence on the cases officially tabulated. Community-wide surveys always find disturbed individuals who are maintaining a marginal social existence; they indicate that statistics based only on hospital and clinic records underestimate the actual prevalence of mental disorders in the general population. A person is as likely to seek psychiatric help because of a family crisis, an economic misfortune or a chance encounter with a public agency as because of the nature of his disorder. Thus single, divorced, widowed or otherwise isolated persons are more likely to be hospitalized than those with family support. Life stress as a precipitant of perceived illness and prolonged hospitalization is a phenomenon of medical and surgical, as well as mental, illnesses.

With medical progress disorders once crudely lumped together as insanity have been separated into discrete entities. One type of insanity, a dementia accompanied by general paralysis, is now known to be the result of pathological changes in the central nervous system caused by the spirochete of syphilis; it can be prevented by the effective treatment of primary syphilis. The complex of mental disturbances associated with pellagra was shown to be the result of a dietary deficiency of B-complex vitamins (tryptophan, nicotinic acid and pyridoxine). Similar disturbances in the absence of dietary inadequacy have now been shown to be the result of an inherited metabolic defect (Hartnup's disease) that leads to an inability to absorb tryptophan from the gut.

The fact that the remedies for schizophrenia and manic-depressive disorders are different has given added significance to the diagnostic differentiation of the two. Studies have shown that American and British psychiatrists have tended to make quite different diagnoses when they are given the same set of symptoms for disorders that could be schizophrenic or manic-depressive. A joint American-British diagnostic study has made it evident that the term schizophrenia has been used much more broadly by American psychiatrists. With more precise attention to the details of the psychiatric examination, because of the therapeutic importance of the diagnostic differentiation, higher degrees of replicability among psychiatrists can be attained. As long as we must rely on clinical judgments made by psychiatrists, in contrast to more objective laboratory indicators, differences of opinion will be inevitable.

It is these characteristics of a mental disorder—its changing definitions, the variability of its course, its responsiveness to the social environment and imprecision in its diagnosis—that make psychiatry a center of controversy. If the recognition and appropriate treatment of psychosis can benefit the afflicted, it is also true that error can harm them. Hospitalization, particularly when it is involuntary, deprives the patient of his personal liberties. It can be misused by civil authorities and by disaffected families to remove unwanted persons from the community.

In the past five years commitment laws in many states have been rewritten to protect civil rights, but the laws will be only as effective as the vigilance of the community, the courts and physicians guarantees. There is, however, a nagging question that should not be forgotten: Are we legislating a justification for indifference to human welfare? If we wish to avoid a paternalistic society, must we settle for an atomistic one? When someone is grossly disturbed but refuses to seek help, what is our responsibility toward him? The law recognizes the legitimacy of intervention when the patient is suicidal or homicidal. Under what other circumstances is intervention warranted? That is a major issue for parents with a disturbed adolescent, for children with a disturbed parent and for friends helplessly watching a life being wasted. It may be that such casualties are the necessary price for the benefits of individual freedom, but the matter deserves more thought than it is being given.

Current psychiatric knowledge is compatible with a stress-diathesis model for the genesis of psychoses: Psychobiological stress acts on an individual with a genetic predisposition to psychosis and eventually leads to abnormal metabolic processes that cause disorders of mood and thought. Predisposition probably varies on a continuum. Although genetic factors are a prerequisite, it is unlikely that they are sufficient to evoke psychosis in themselves. The behavior of the mentally disturbed person may cause others to reject him, so that he experiences additional severe psychological stress.

At any given time the power of psychiatric remedies and their accessibility to the patient are major determinants of the outcome of an acute mental breakdown. Therapeutic drugs not only presumably restore metabolic equilibrium but also may directly affect the patient's perception of stress. The probability of further personality deterioration and the duration of the disorder is a function of the social environment provided for the patient by the health-care system. The degree of organization or disorganization of the community where a psychotic person finds himself will influence his mood and thought directly.

Our ability to identify the significant psychobiological stressors is limited, and it is still not possible to estimate degrees of genetic predisposition accurately enough to take preventive measures. There have nonetheless been major advances in our capacity for controlling or aborting mental disorders when they do occur. Moreover, we appear to be on the verge of answering some of the basic questions about the functioning of the brain. Psychiatric research is a fragile enterprise, yet it is currently argued in ruling Government circles that it should receive not more public support but less. It would be the height of folly to stifle fundamental investigation just at the time when it holds so much promise for revealing the basic mechanisms of psychotic disorders and for developing rational therapies aimed at the causes of psychoses and not merely at their symptoms.

IX

The Hospital

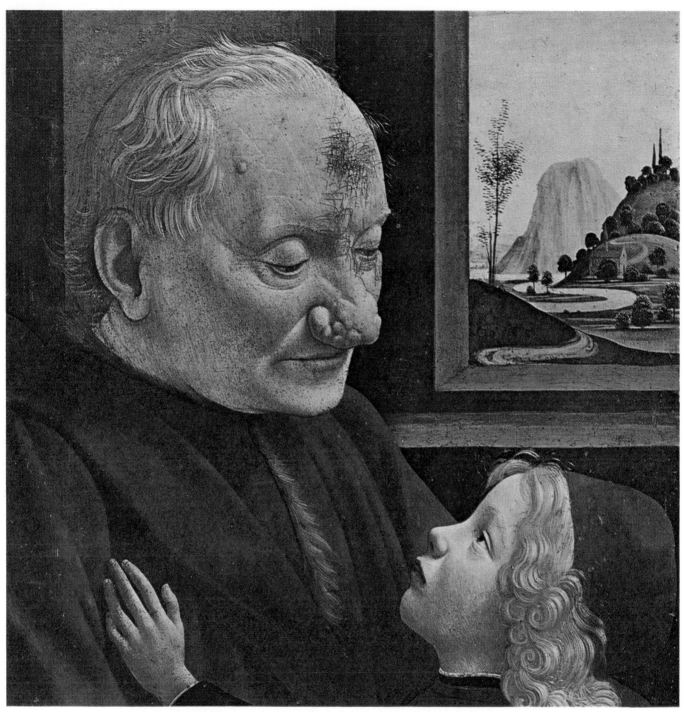

The painting shown here symbolizes the theme of this volume: life and death and
medicine. It is a reproduction of *An Old Man and His Grandson,* painted by Domen-
ico Ghirlandaio late in the 15th century, which hangs in the Louvre. The painting is
notable for its affecting representation of the family relationship, of the contrast of
unblemished childhood with old age and sickness and of the child's uncomprehend-
ing acceptance of his grandfather's disfigurement. The old man apparently suffers
from rhinophyma, a condition in which the nose becomes knobby and enlarged as a
result of rosacea, a chronic disease involving overactivity of the sebaceous glands.
Usually the nose is also reddened, because small blood vessels become dilated. The
reason it is not depicted as red may be that it was not red when Ghirlandaio saw the
old man: this portrait was based on a drawing that Ghirlandaio had done of the old
man on his deathbed after his death. (Courtesy of the Bettmann Archive, Inc.)

The Hospital

JOHN H. KNOWLES

It is increasingly where the patient sees the physician. It brings together the specialists, structures their collaboration, provides their supporting personnel and supplies materials and machines

There are wide differences among the hospitals of the U.S. depending on their size, their type of sponsorship (voluntary, proprietary or government), their provision of services (general as contrasted with specialty services such as mental, eye, obstetrical or pediatric) and the nature of their affiliation (university teaching as contrasted with community, nonaffiliated hospitals). Regardless of their differences, they exemplify man's perpetual struggle against disease and suffering.

In its present form the hospital has been shaped by the needs of society and reflects not only its attitudes, beliefs and values but also its economy. In the past half-century scientific and technological developments have contributed so heavily to the diagnosis, treatment and prevention of disease that it is no longer possible for the physician to work effectively without the modern apparatus and the specialists and technicians centralized in the hospital. As in so much of modern institutional and technology-based life, the threat of dehumanization of personal relationships—here between the physician and the patient—has in many instances become a reality.

The fact remains that the steady expansion of knowledge has necessitated specialization and the housing of advanced technology within the walls of the modern hospital and that these developments have been of pronounced benefit to mankind. Progress in medical science and in the specialized division of medical skills has changed medicine from an individual, intuitive enterprise into a social service. The hospital is the institutional form of this social service. It has evolved from a house of despair for the sick poor to a house of hope for all social and economic classes in just the past 60 years.

The earliest hospitals were the healing temples of ancient Egypt, the public hospitals of Buddhist India and the Muslim East and the sick houses (Beit Holem) of Israel. The ancient Oriental custom of providing hospitality for guests and travelers pervaded the lands of the eastern Mediterranean, and houses were built where weary travelers and strangers could stop for food, lodging and, if they were sick, for nursing care. The derivation of the word "hospital" shows what an important part these travelers and their hosts played in the evolution of the hospital. "Hospital" comes from the Latin *hospes,* meaning host or guest. The English word comes from the medieval Latin *hospitale,* as do "hostel" and "hotel." "Hospital," "hostel" and "hotel" were at one time used interchangeably.

The evolution of the modern hospital is usually associated with the advent of Christianity. The Christian ethic of faith, humanitarianism and charity resulted in the establishment of a vast hospital system. At the Council of Nicaea in A.D. 325 the bishops were instructed to establish hospitals in every cathedral city. Constantine I, the first of the Roman emperors to embrace Christianity, ordered the closing of all pagan temples of healing in A.D. 335.

During the great Crusades between 1096 and 1291 numerous hostels for the sick were established along the way to the Holy Land. In England, St. Bartholomew's and St. Thomas's hospitals were founded by monks in 1123 and 1215. Medicine was practiced by monks and priests in the hostels adjacent to the monasteries or in designated areas of the monasteries. Peripatetic apothecaries and blood-letting surgeons plied their trade in the homes of their patients. Only the destitute, weary travelers and those with diseases regarded as hopeless found their way to the hospitals. When the parliament of Henry VIII suppressed the monastery system of England between 1536 and 1539, the hospital system disappeared with it. St. Bartholomew's and St. Thomas's were refounded on a secular basis; the two hospitals cared for the entire sick population of London for the next 170 years. Where the monastery system had cared for the incurable, the sick poor and those with specific disabilities (such as the lame, the blind, the aged, lepers and orphans), the burden of patients forced the London hospitals to limit their work to the curable sick. In 1700 the orders of St. Thomas's recorded: "No incurables are to be received." It was the first time in Western history that the hospital had taken up an active, curative role in medical care. This in turn accelerated the development of the almshouse for the care of incurables.

During the 18th century most of the care given in hospitals was nursing. The hospital remained an institution for the sick poor. The Hôtel-Dieu, founded by the bishop of Paris, probably in the seventh century, and the oldest hospital in existence today, had some 2,000 beds. In 1788 the death rate among its patients was nearly 25 percent, and frequently two and sometimes eight patients occupied one bed. It was also noted that attendants living in the hospital had a death rate of 6 to 12 percent per year. It was not until 1793 that the National Convention of the French Revolution ruled that there should be only one patient to a bed and that the beds should be separated by at least three feet.

Not until late in the 19th century could hospitals be said to benefit any substantial number of patients. When Florence Nightingale returned from the

Crimean War (where she had demonstrated the marked reduction in morbidity and mortality that could be brought about by improved nursing practices), she wrote: "The very first requirement in a hospital [is] that it should do the sick no harm."

With the growth of private philanthropy in the 18th century the first voluntary (privately endowed) hospitals were established. Thomas Guy, a wealthy London merchant, founded the hospital bearing his name in 1721. In the 19th century teaching hospitals were founded in England that served as the prototype of the voluntary hospitals that ultimately arose in America.

The most powerful stimulus to the evolution of the American hospital was the growth of the cities. Urbanization concentrated the need for care and provided the talents and facilities for the solution of the problem. This stimulus and the medical profession's need for

teaching and research facilities led to the founding of voluntary urban teaching hospitals. New York Hospital, chartered in 1771, was affiliated with Columbia University and later with the Cornell University Medical College (1927). The Massachusetts General Hospital was founded in 1811; it is affiliated with the Harvard Medical School. In Canada the Montreal General Hospital was founded in 1821; its medical staff became the faculty of the first Canadian medical school, established by McGill University in 1829. Today most urban hospitals, whether voluntary or under municipal or state control, are affiliated with universities and their medical schools. They have a wide variety of teaching and research functions in addition to their primary function of patient care.

The American hospital did not assume its present form until this century. Hospital architecture reflected the fact

that only the sick poor came to hospitals and also the main danger of hospitalization: "hospitalism," or cross infection among patients. Hospital wards were large pavilions built in blockhouse style for maximum cross ventilation and sunlight and allowed for the wide separation of beds, which might number as many as 40. Louis Pasteur's demonstration that disease was caused by microbes and that microbes could be destroyed by heat stimulated Joseph Lister, professor of surgery at Glasgow, to develop antiseptic techniques in surgery. Hospitalism diminished, but it was not until the introduction of sulfanilamide in the mid-1930's and of penicillin in the early 1940's that this scourge abated sufficiently to allow surgery without prohibitive morbidity and mortality due to infection. To this day, however, hospital-acquired infections, now from antibiotic-resistant organisms, remain a problem.

The use of ether as an anesthetic agent

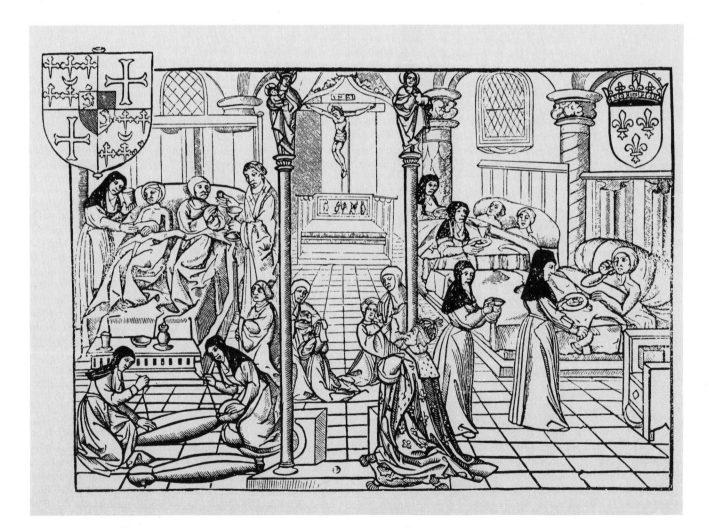

HOSPITALITY FOR THE SICK was the function of the Hôtel-Dieu of Paris, a hospital probably founded in the seventh century and today the largest in the city. When this 16th-century wood engraving was made, and indeed until the 20th century, hospitals cared mainly for the poor and for transients, and their services were limited to bed and board and rudimentary nursing. The man attending the bed at left is not a physician but a priest serving the Eucharist. Other patients are served by nuns; at left two more nuns sew shrouds. That some beds were occupied by more than one patient was not unusual; the practice continued until 1793.

was first demonstrated at the Massachusetts General Hospital in 1846 by W. T. G. Morton. It proved to be a tremendous stimulus to the development of surgery. Until decades thereafter blood transfusion, now so necessary for the well-being of the patient in many forms of surgery, was hazardous at best. The discovery of blood groups and their incompatibility by Karl Landsteiner in 1900 and the first use of sodium citrate in 1913 to prevent clotting made it possible to give lifesaving transfusions without disaster. Storage of blood then became possible, but the full development of blood banks (with refrigerated blood) in hospitals did not come until well into the 1930's. Until that time "fresh" donors were bled and the blood was transfused while it was still warm.

When W. K. Röntgen described his "new kind of rays" in 1895, the modern technology of radiology (or roentgenology) and radiotherapy was born. By 1896 X rays were used in the diagnosis of bone fractures and dislocations. By the early 1900's most of the major urban hospitals in the U.S. had installed X-ray machines, and by 1915 most had established separate departments of radiology. The use of barium salts allowed visualization of the gastrointestinal tract, and by the 1930's a wide variety of radio-opaque materials made possible the X-ray visualization of practically all the organ systems of the body: bronchopulmonary, genitourinary, cerebrospinal and vascular. This allowed accurate diagnosis of a wide variety of diseases and injuries and gave further stimulus to the transformation of the hospital from a passive receptacle for the sick poor to an active caring institution for all social and economic classes. Hospital architecture began to change to accommodate the new technology. Single rooms for the affluent were established in the 1910's and 1920's, and two-to-four-bed ("semiprivate") rooms were installed in the 1920's and 1930's.

In the 1940's and 1950's the American hospital underwent an even more dramatic transformation. The intensive use of antibiotics meant that infections no longer claimed the lives of the elderly, so that more of the hospital's resources could be used for the diagnosis and treatment of the chronic degenerative diseases of old age: cancer, heart disease and stroke, arthritis and emphysema. Today more than a fourth of all money spent on health in the U.S. (including payments for hospitals, physicians, drugs and extended-care services) is spent on

the tenth of our population who are 65 or older. Antibiotics have also markedly diminished the need for pediatric and infectious-disease hospital facilities and freed beds for the diagnosis and treatment of children with congenital diseases and deformities, behavioral problems and accidents. Streptomycin and isoniazid have diminished the need for state tuberculosis sanatoriums. They have either been closed as the need for bed rest and hospitalization in the treatment of tuberculosis has waned or have been used for the increasing numbers of patients with chest diseases such as chronic bronchitis and emphysema.

The care of the mentally ill in distant upland sanatoriums and state asylums has similarly been transformed by the intensive use of psychoactive drugs and the development of a "positive" therapeutic environment (as contrasted with the traditional "passive" custodial function) and "halfway" houses [see "Psychiatric Intervention," by Leon Eisenberg, page 79]. This has reduced the length of stay in mental institutions while markedly increasing the discharge rate of patients back to the community: from 35 per 100 admitted in 1920 to 85 per 100 by 1953. At the same time "acute" urban general hospitals have developed facilities for the short-term care of acute psychiatric illness.

As chronic illness (mental and degenerative disease such as heart disease, cancer, stroke, arthritis, chronic bronchitis and emphysema) has increased in an expanding population of elderly people, the need to develop and enlarge ambulatory and rehabilitation facilities has been met by many hospitals. By the same token hospitals for the care of the chronically ill, bedridden patient have been found to be in short supply, and the existing ones (usually built and managed by state governments but in some instances operated under religious auspices) are frequently understaffed and underfinanced. Extended-care facilities and nursing homes for the care of the chronically ill have been developed largely under proprietary auspices and in many regions of the U.S. they either are substandard or do not have enough beds for the task. As a result many patients are kept in high-cost acute hospital beds when the use of lower-cost facilities is indicated.

Following World War II the centripetal effects of a rapidly expanding medical technology that could be based only in the hospital and an increasing utilization of physicians by a steadily expanding population pushed both the patient

and the physician closer to the hospital. Because of the maldistribution and apparent shortage of overworked physicians, and because of the real limitations of the house call, the patient and the physician turned increasingly in time of need to the ambulatory clinic and the emergency ward of the urban hospital. The emergency ward became what the church had been in the Middle Ages: a sanctuary for those with any form of disease—social, psychic or somatic. Not only is there an ever increasing number of accidents (largely related to alcohol and the automobile) and somatic crises such as heart attacks and strokes, but also more and more people are using the hospital's emergency facilities for social and psychological problems: alcoholics and narcotic addicts, people in acute anxiety states, attempted suicides, people with venereal disease and people in crisis situations such as loss of a job or a death in the family.

As health was perceived more and more as a birthright rather than a privilege, access to high-quality care for all Americans was demanded. Ambulatory clinics and emergency wards were expanded. Outpatient visits increased from 65 million in 1954 to more than 180 million in 1970. Visits to physicians in hospitals as a fraction of all physician visits increased from 10.2 percent to 21.1 percent, that is, one in every five physician-patient encounters now takes place in a hospital.

Meanwhile urban hospitals expanded or were rebuilt to meet the increasing needs and demands of the expanding population. Scientific and technological advances stimulated the need for new surgical facilities and the development of intensive-care units, complete with electronic monitoring devices, specialist nurses and technicians. Thoracic surgery developed rapidly during both world wars; the first pneumonectomy (removal of an entire lung) and lobectomy (removal of a lobe of the lung) were accomplished in the 1930's. Cardiac catheterization and angiography (the use of a hollow tube threaded through an arm vein and into the heart with the injection of radio-opaque dye for the X-ray visualization of lung and heart vessels and valves) developed rapidly in the 1940's and made possible accurate diagnosis of congenital and acquired heart disease (largely valvular deformities due to rheumatic fever). That ushered in a new era of cardiac and vascular surgery. The modern era of "spare parts" surgery began with the first successful transplantation of a kidney in 1954 and with the development of prosthetic devices such as artificial heart valves and artificial blood vessels with which to replace diseased, worn-out or injured ones.

These developments, along with an increasing demand for surgery in cancer and in the correction of injuries and deformities of all parts of the body, have transformed the urban general hospital into a highly technical, high-cost, acute curative institution in which perhaps as much as 70 percent of the facilities and personnel are today related to the care of surgical patients. Scientific and technological developments have necessitated specialization for all health professionals, whether they are physicians, nurses or technicians. Intensive-care units for patients with heart attacks, strokes, severe injuries, neonatal disease,

chronic lung disease, acute infections resistant to antibiotics, and burns have concentrated specialists and their technology in specific areas of the hospital. These units have largely evolved only in the past 10 years. They cost as much as $500 per day per patient to operate. Today there are more than 50 job descriptions in the personnel office of the urban general hospital. As the subdivision of labor increases, the difficulty of organizing such a diverse group increases. Efficiency falters, costs increase and the atomized, fragmented "machine" approach to the patient dehumanizes what should be an intensely personal and humane encounter. On balance, however, it can be stated that the benefits of modern medicine far outweigh the drawbacks.

Like everything else in our pluralistic country the diversity of hospitals defies

simple description. The Federal Government operates a wide variety of hospitals: through the Department of Defense for servicemen and their dependents, the Veterans Administration for the care of veterans with both service- and non-service-connected disabilities, and the Department of Health, Education, and Welfare for American Indians, Alaskan natives, narcotic addicts, lepers and Federal employees injured on the job. Non-Federal, government-controlled hospitals include some 2,000 municipal, county and district hospitals. The New York City Health and Hospitals Corporation operates 19 municipal hospitals with 15,000 beds; they provide care for more than 1.5 million medically indigent New Yorkers and employ more than 40,000 people with an annual payroll of $400 million. Contrast this large urban hospi-

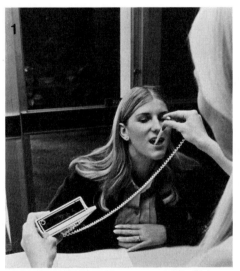 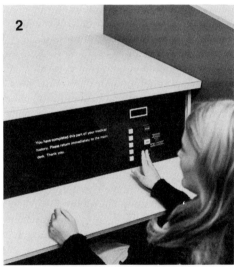 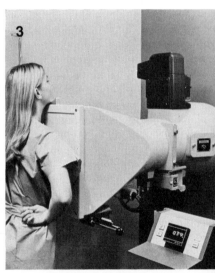

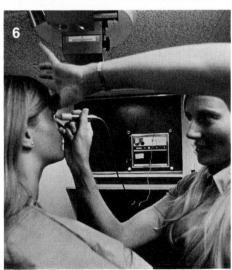 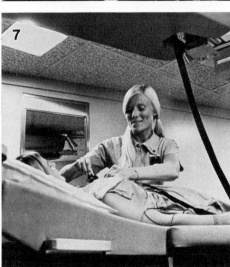 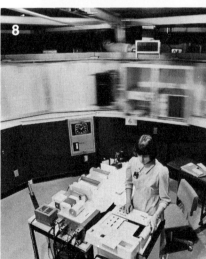

AUTOMATED MULTIPHASIC LABORATORY at the Palo Alto Medical Clinic in Palo Alto, Calif., represents one application of new technology to hospital practice. The laboratory, which processes test results by computer, is used for periodic physical checkups and for examinations prior to hospital admission. The patient first has her temperature electronically recorded (1) and

drinks a glucose solution at the registration desk. She reports her medical history in conversation with a computer (2). About 900 questions are filed in a "branching logic" film memory; an affirmative response to a general inquiry may call up more specific related questions. After completing the medical-history questionnaire the patient puts on a disposable paper gown and slippers. Her weight

tal system with the 3,500 U.S. hospitals having fewer than 100 beds that represent the majority of the proprietary (profit-making) hospitals. (We are, in fact, a nation of small hospitals.)

Certain characteristics and trends in the decade from 1961 to 1971 are notable:

1. The number of hospitals has increased because of the construction of larger government (non-Federal) short-stay hospitals. Even though nongovernment hospitals decreased in number, the absolute number of beds under these auspices increased.

2. Long-term hospitals have decreased in number (and this fact is responsible for an overall decrease in hospital beds), partly reflecting a profound change in the treatment of certain diseases (tu-berculosis, mental illness) but, more important, indicating a lack of interest in much-needed hospital facilities for the chronically ill, bedridden patient. This is highly undesirable from the standpoint not only of quality of care but also of cost. Many such patients have to be sustained in higher-cost, acute hospital facilities.

3. The number of general hospitals has increased and the number of specialty hospitals has declined. This is highly desirable. Specialty hospitals, unless they are immediately adjacent to general hospitals, simply cannot provide the comprehensive services that are necessary to the complete care of the patient.

4. Smaller hospitals have declined in number as the desirable trend to larger, general hospitals has accelerated.

5. Intensive-care units (particularly those for patients with heart attacks) have proliferated rapidly. So have psychiatric inpatient services. The latter trend reflects both the increase in acute mental and social illness and the movement to integrate the care of patients with psychiatric disorders into the urban general hospital and out of the isolated, distant asylum.

6. The development of hospital family-planning services bespeaks recognition of the undesirability of unwanted pregnancies. Similarly, a decrease in the number of maternity hospitals reflects the decrease in the birthrate and widespread public acceptance of smaller families.

7. An increase in hospital social-work departments recognizes the highly complex social and economic problems surrounding illness, and the need of the patient for help in reordering this environment for his best care.

8. As the total number of hospital beds decreased and admissions and length of stay increased, the average occupancy rate fell, indicating a suboptimal utilization of high-cost hospital facilities. Overall, I believe we remain overbedded in the U.S., which means we are underutilizing high-cost facilities and are therefore contributing to unnecessary expense.

9. More than 2.5 million people were employed full time in hospitals in 1971. Their payroll accounted for 60 percent of total hospital expenses. In addition another 500,000 people were employed part time. The health field in general is rapidly becoming the largest "industry" in the U.S. as we change from an industrial economy to a service one. The majority of health workers are employed by hospitals. The marked increase in the number of employees per hospital bed over the decade reflects the scientific and technical complexities of modern medical care that have occasioned the increasing subdivision of technical work and increased numbers of technical workers. The development of intensive-care units is a case in point. The marked increase in the average salary reflects both the imbalance of supply and demand for health workers and, more important, the highly desirable increased value placed on such workers. Service workers generally (for example teachers and letter carriers) gained marked increases in pay and fringe benefits in the decade of the 1960's. The union movement obtained a strong foothold in hospitals and accelerated the trend toward more equitable treatment of hospital employees.

10. The number of hospitals affiliated with medical schools has increased

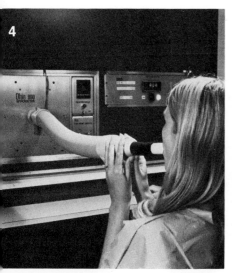
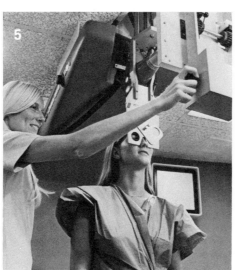
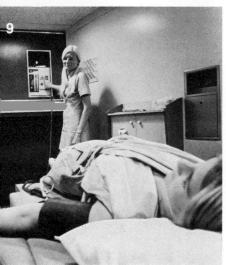
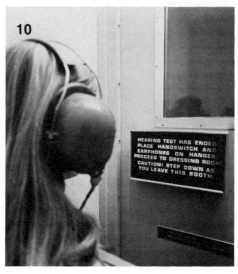

and height are recorded automatically and an X-ray photograph of her chest is made (*3*). She then enters a room in the "carousel," where several more tests are performed. These include spirometry (*4*), near and distant vision (*5*), tonometry (*6*) and electrocardiography (*7*). The recorder for this last test is in the core of the carousel (*8*), where revolving walls bring instruments to each test room. Blood pressure is monitored electronically (*9*) and hearing is tested in a soundproof cubicle (*10*). The procedure takes two hours and costs $55.

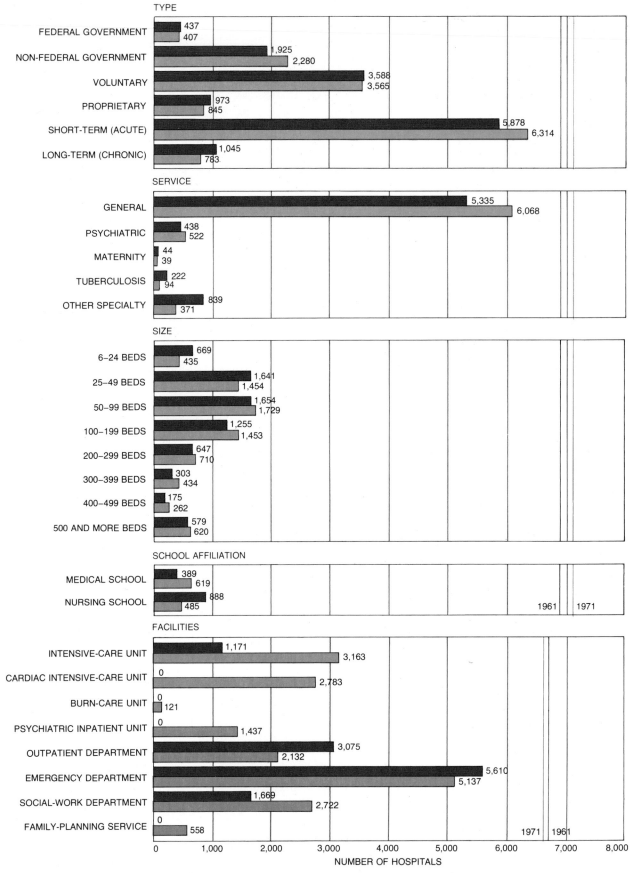

TYPE

FEDERAL GOVERNMENT	437 / 407
NON-FEDERAL GOVERNMENT	1,925 / 2,280
VOLUNTARY	3,588 / 3,565
PROPRIETARY	973 / 845
SHORT-TERM (ACUTE)	5,878 / 6,314
LONG-TERM (CHRONIC)	1,045 / 783

SERVICE

GENERAL	5,335 / 6,068
PSYCHIATRIC	438 / 522
MATERNITY	44 / 39
TUBERCULOSIS	222 / 94
OTHER SPECIALTY	839 / 371

SIZE

6–24 BEDS	669 / 435
25–49 BEDS	1,641 / 1,454
50–99 BEDS	1,654 / 1,729
100–199 BEDS	1,255 / 1,453
200–299 BEDS	647 / 710
300–399 BEDS	303 / 434
400–499 BEDS	175 / 262
500 AND MORE BEDS	579 / 620

SCHOOL AFFILIATION

MEDICAL SCHOOL	389 / 619
NURSING SCHOOL	888 / 485

1961   1971

FACILITIES

INTENSIVE-CARE UNIT	1,171 / 3,163
CARDIAC INTENSIVE-CARE UNIT	0 / 2,783
BURN-CARE UNIT	0 / 121
PSYCHIATRIC INPATIENT UNIT	0 / 1,437
OUTPATIENT DEPARTMENT	3,075 / 2,132
EMERGENCY DEPARTMENT	5,610 / 5,137
SOCIAL-WORK DEPARTMENT	1,669 / 2,722
FAMILY-PLANNING SERVICE	0 / 558

1971   1961

0   1,000   2,000   3,000   4,000   5,000   6,000   7,000   8,000
NUMBER OF HOSPITALS

THE LARGE GENERAL HOSPITAL for the short-term care of the acutely ill appears to be growing faster than all other types of hospital in graphs derived from data compiled by the American Hospital Association for the years 1961 (*gray*) and 1971 (*color*). The influence of technology and the broadening of hospital services are suggested by the growth of intensive-care units, social-work departments and other specialized facilities. An apparent decline in outpatient clinics and emergency rooms is caused in part by changes in reporting procedures. Vertical lines at 6,923 and 7,097 indicate the total number of hospitals in the U.S. in 1961 and 1971 respectively. In tabulations of hospital facilities only institutions that responded to the survey are included. For those graphs the totals are 6,712 hospitals in 1961 and 6,622 in 1971. Most of the hospital building was done by state and municipal governments.

markedly. The best medical care is achieved in an environment of constant inquiry and scrutiny by a number of people (medical students, house-staff interns and residents, senior-staff professors and practicing physicians), where scientific and technical knowledge can be applied within the shortest period of time after its development. Equally important, the teaching hospitals provide for tomorrow's health needs by the training of physicians, nurses and other health workers through practical, supervised experience. Ideally all hospitals should be affiliated with medical schools, but this is not possible, at least at the moment; physicians practicing in the community steadfastly resist the controls inherent in medical-school affiliation. Most teaching hospitals are large and in an urban location adjacent to the university's medical school. Although only 619 of the nation's 7,097 hospitals are affiliated, they represent about half of the nation's hospital beds. Interns and residents account for about 15 percent of the nation's practicing physicians. Their services are essential to the hospital's patients. Some 35 percent of the interns and residents are recruited from abroad, where their training is generally inferior to that received in American medical schools. Many of these foreign medical graduates work in community and state institutions, where the quality of the care they give may be poor.

11. The number of hospitals that operate schools of nursing has decreased precipitously as the drive to gain full professional status for nurses has fostered the development of schools of nursing within colleges and universities. I believe there is a need for both the diploma (hospital) school and the baccalaureate programs. A balance of these interests should be maintained.

No account of American hospitals would be complete without a discussion of hospital costs. In 1925 the cost of one day's hospitalization at the Massachusetts General Hospital was $3. The bill was paid directly by the patient out of his own pocket, and he stayed for 15 days for a total cost of $56.20. In 1972 a patient would stay for an average of seven days at a total cost of $1,400, and the bill would be paid by any one of a variety of third parties. Indeed, between 1962 and 1972 the percent of hospital income from patients paying directly declined from 38 percent to 12 percent. In the same decade income from the Blue Cross and state welfare departments increased, and Medicare (instituted in 1966) assumed 27 percent of hospital income. At the same time the continued decline of endowment income in covering the cost of free care confirms the unpleasant truth that voluntary hospitals can no longer assume the ultimate responsibility for their economic lifeline. That responsibility must be assumed by the community's (and the nation's) public and private agencies.

Where does the money go? Hospital inpatient costs are categorized under "routine" costs and ancillary expense. When the citizen hears that "routine" room-and-board costs are $92 a day, he is staggered and may demand that he be cared for in a hotel. He does not realize that room and board includes (1) 50 different diets of three meals a day served in bed (sometimes six for ulcer patients and diabetics), (2) the salaries of three shifts of nurses per day seven days a week, (3) the salaries of house staff (interns and residents) available to the patient 24 hours a day and (4) the cost of supplies, medical records and medical social workers. The comparable hotel costs in the hospital come to about $23 per day, which compares favorably with costs in the hotel industry.

When one adds the ancillary costs, the average total cost (at the Massachusetts General Hospital in 1972) was $170.45 per day. Ancillary expense includes operating rooms, laboratories, medical supplies and drugs, radiology and anesthesiology—much of which the patient never sees. It is small wonder that almost everyone complains about hospital costs when there is no valid comparison with any other known experience and almost no one tries to find out exactly what is included in the cost of a one-day stay in a hospital.

The bill for staying in a teaching hospital is higher than that for staying in a community hospital because of the added cost of training nurses, physicians and other health workers, and because of the higher cost of caring for patients with complex illnesses referred to the urban medical center. It is worth mentioning that a man suffering a heart attack in 1920 would have stayed for as long as eight weeks at the Massachusetts General Hospital for a total cost of $180, that in 1930 he would have stayed six weeks for $210 and that in 1970 he would have stayed four weeks for $3,500 (which would have included $1,500 for 10 days in the intensive-care unit and $2,000 for 20 days in a regular bed). Of 100 men treated for heart attacks in 1920, however, 40 died; of 100 treated in 1930, 30 died, and of 100 treated in 1970 only 18 died. The benefit of 22 additional live men per 100 in 1970—men who could go back to work, raise their families, add to the gross national product and pay their taxes—more than justifies the cost.

Having noted these benefits, we must also recognize the marked inflation of medical-care costs over the past 20 years, fueled particularly by the advent of Medicare in 1966. For the three years from June, 1966, to June, 1969, the consumer price index rose 13 percent; prices for medical care rose 22.2 percent. Hospital daily service charges increased 54.6 percent; physicians' fees increased 21.5 percent. Price controls were inevitable. The Administration moved to institute its Economic Stabilization Program, now in Phase 4.

What can be done to contain hospital costs? The full and appropriate utilization of hospital beds is the single most important factor in holding down costs. Management techniques to ensure vastly improved cost accounting are needed by many hospitals. One cannot control costs when they are not identifiable and quantifiable. Turnover rates of hospital employees must be reduced. (For example, it may cost between $1,000 and $2,000 to bring a new nurse to fully effective performance, and present turnover rates are as high as 70 percent per year in American hospitals.) Other management techniques to reduce overtime, to improve working conditions and to make maximal use of industrial engineers, systems analysts, automatic machines and computers can help to keep costs down.

All of this is required in the management of hospitals, but factors external to the hospital will do far more to reduce the national expenditure for hospital services. Regional planning is needed to ensure the full utilization of facilities and to avoid the duplication of costly services. (Vascular surgery and the radioactive-cobalt treatment of cancer are cases in point.) Dramatic changes in health insurance are needed to favor lower-cost services, health education and preventive-medicine programs, to provide incentives for improved management and to enforce rigid quality controls. Finally, far more group, prepaid comprehensive medical-care programs (such as the Kaiser-Permanente system) should be developed. The reduction in unnecessary surgery and hospitalization under such systems is dramatic. The physician can be the prime mover in developments of this kind, but all too often he and the American Medical Association have been the prime resisters.

Although almost all Americans are

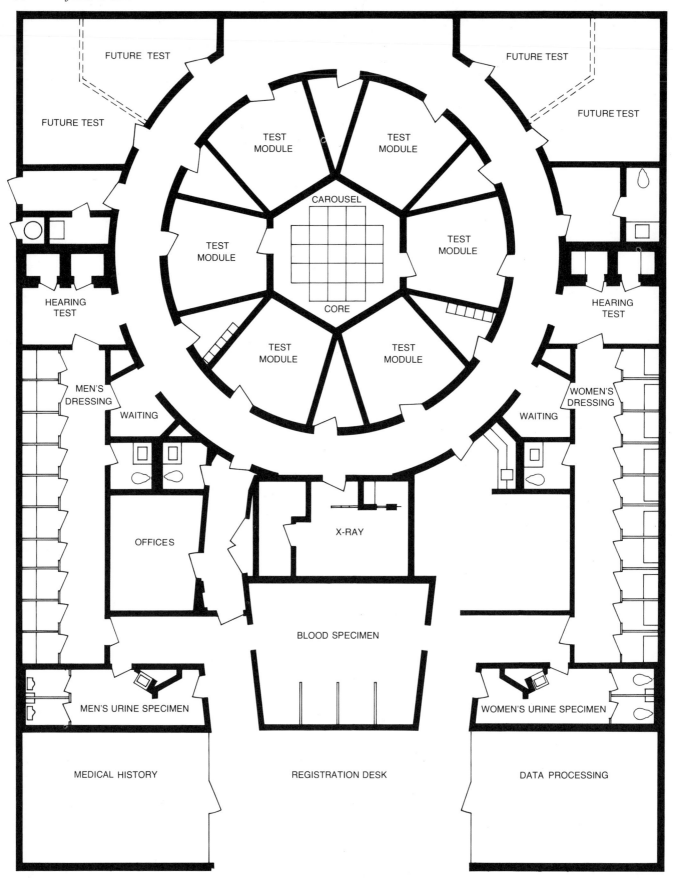

CAROUSEL SURROUNDED BY TEST MODULES forms the heart of the Palo Alto Clinic's Automated Multiphasic Laboratory. The carousel is the hexagonal structure near the top. Every five minutes a three-foot-high section of its walls revolves 60 degrees, bringing new instruments to each of the six test rooms. Thus every half-hour each room has access to all the instruments. Some expensive devices, such as electrocardiogram recorders, are housed in the core of the carousel and connected in turn to each patient. Certain tests, such as X rays and audiograms, are performed in other areas of the laboratory; the computer-administered medical-history questionnaire is answered in the room at left at the bottom of the diagram. One technician stays with the patient through most of the procedure. Test results are delivered to the attending physician as a computer printout. The design of the laboratory is patented.

aware of the unique contributions American medicine has made to their welfare, the cost of hospitalization has become an increasing source of frustration and outright anger to many. Rising expectations have been matched by rising costs. In the new age of the consumer, demands for public accountability have increased and resulted in the establishment of state rate-review agencies, in more assiduous attempts on the part of third-party payers to control hospital costs and in the passage of state laws that require certificates of need before hospital construction can proceed. Increasingly hospitals are subject to the kind of regulation and control that has been applied to public utilities.

The roles of the hospital trustee, the hospital physician and the hospital administrator are being seriously questioned. Have trustees really exercised their full responsibility for prudent management and the regional planning of hospitals? The physician has the ultimate authority in the use of the hospital, but has he exercised his full responsibility for efficient management, for the best use of the facilities and, again, for regional planning? The hospital is almost unique among contemporary institutions in the number of powerful outside forces that exercise control over various aspects of the hospital's life, and one wonders how many hospital trustees understand these complexities. State departments of public health inspect and license hospitals, usually on a biannual basis, looking at everything from the safety of X-ray machines to the cleanliness of operating rooms. The Joint Commission on Accreditation of Hospitals (with membership from the American Medical Association, the American Hospital Association, the American College of Physicians and the American College of Surgeons) conducts its own (usually more rigorous) inspection of hospitals every two years, in some instances duplicating the work of the state. Blue Cross associations are beginning to insist on regional planning, on the increased use of lower-cost ambulatory facilities and on more stringent cost, quality and utilization controls before contracting with or reimbursing the hospital. As hospitals do their best to serve the indigent sick, state welfare departments delay the processing and payment of claims, causing the hospitals to complain bitterly when their receivables mount. The steadily proliferating state review boards for hospital reimbursement and hospital planning have struggled, often inefficiently, to enforce regional planning and to contain costs.

The A.M.A., through its Council on Medical Education and Hospitals, accredits the intern and residency programs of the teaching hospitals. Nineteen national specialty boards set their own requirements for hospital training and experience, generally in isolation from one another and with no apparent reference to the national need for various types of specialists. For example, there is in the U.S. an excess of general surgeons and neurosurgeons and a severe shortage of anesthesiologists and pediatric psychiatrists. Yet internships and residency programs are filled to overflowing with the former, and the well for the latter is nearly dry. In addition to the various professional medical unions, labor unions have gained a powerful voice in the control of the hospital and its policies.

The Federal Government, through a wide variety of programs (for example Medicare and the Hill-Burton Act), sets requirements for utilization of hospitals and its own unique reimbursement formulas (which are different from the state Medicaid formulas). Federal research funds, largely from the National Institutes of Health, for those affiliated teaching hospitals that conduct such programs impose another set of controls and requirements on the hospital. Over a 12-month period the teaching hospital may be audited by as many as five different public and private agencies, in addition to the auditors who report to its own board of trustees.

Finally, the teaching hospital has to balance the long-term needs of the university—indeed, of the community—for teaching and research with the immediate needs of the community for care. The two needs are frequently in conflict, and when one overwhelms the other, they both suffer. So do the patients! The first function of any hospital worthy of the name is to serve the sick and injured, but the quality of care is highest in an environment of constant intellectual ferment and inquiry. Service and teaching-research are complementary activities, but the balancing act remains a difficult one.

Perhaps the most profound and promising development in the evolution of the American hospital has been its gradual emergence as a health center. Although this potential is far from being realized, the hospital is no longer solely a passive, acute, after-the-fact, curative institution. Through the development of emergency wards, social-service departments and ambulatory clinics, through liaison with extended-care facilities, nursing homes, chronic hospitals and home-care services and through the establishment of neighborhood centers it has extended its interests actively to the community in the interests of keeping down costs, reaching more people in need and preventing, or at least containing, illness. The hospital is, or should be, the community's major institution for the coordination of health planning.

Meanwhile public clamor and political pressure mount for national health insurance, largely owing to the high cost of medical care and an unacceptable level of uneven quality and accessibility of service. The thunder on the right and left becomes deafening as the conservatives call for free-market medicine and the liberals push for the beneficent state. Indeed, the major issue facing hospitals in the 1970's is whether or not we will be able to maintain a voluntary hospital system alongside a public system. Two hundred and twenty years after the founding of Guy's Hospital in London, the forebear of our American voluntary hospital, the British nationalized their health services. The more useful and vital a service becomes in the social order, the more certain it is to be identified with the functions of government. Yet our government's example in the management of its municipal, state and Federal hospitals belies any notion that increasing (or absolute) government control would somehow lead us to a promised land of high quality and accessible health services for all Americans at reasonable cost. I believe we must strengthen both private and public hospitals, ensure standards, quality controls and regional planning through legislation and requirements for reimbursement, and maintain a voluntary hospital system that can guarantee heterodoxy and pluralistic approaches to problem solving. The strength of the American experiment will lie in its ability to balance public and private interest, responsibility to the public good and freedom to enjoy regional self-determination. A complete welfare state will result in a supine citizenry, an erosion of individual initiative and the steady expansion of an inefficient, unresponsive bureaucracy.

Certainly much can and should be done to contain the staggering costs of medical care. Inappropriate, high-cost hospital utilization and appalling amounts of unnecessary surgery cost the American people billions of dollars annually. Part of this is due to ignorance, part to avarice and part to expediency, and the burden of responsibility must rest squarely on the shoulders of the American medical profession. The facts are well established; we need no more

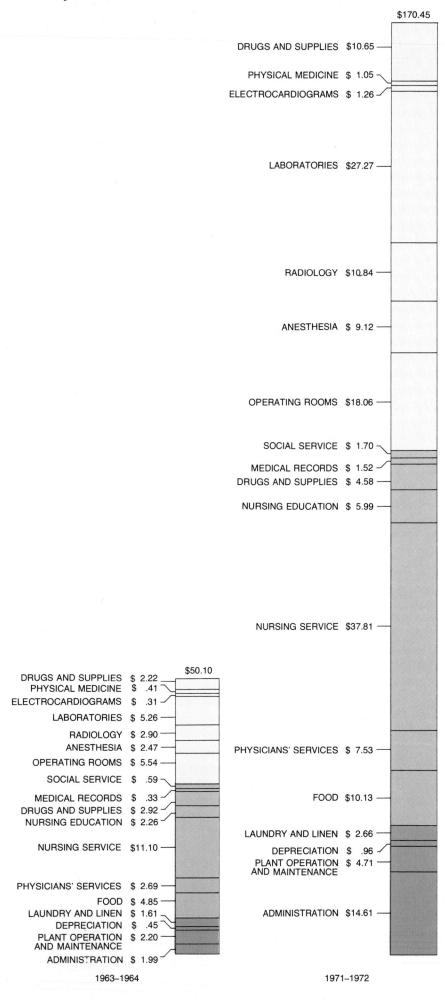

$170.45

DRUGS AND SUPPLIES $10.65

PHYSICAL MEDICINE $ 1.05

ELECTROCARDIOGRAMS $ 1.26

LABORATORIES $27.27

RADIOLOGY $10.84

ANESTHESIA $ 9.12

OPERATING ROOMS $18.06

SOCIAL SERVICE $ 1.70

MEDICAL RECORDS $ 1.52

DRUGS AND SUPPLIES $ 4.58

NURSING EDUCATION $ 5.99

NURSING SERVICE $37.81

PHYSICIANS' SERVICES $ 7.53

FOOD $10.13

LAUNDRY AND LINEN $ 2.66

DEPRECIATION $ .96

PLANT OPERATION $ 4.71
AND MAINTENANCE

ADMINISTRATION $14.61

$50.10

DRUGS AND SUPPLIES $ 2.22
PHYSICAL MEDICINE $ .41
ELECTROCARDIOGRAMS $ .31
LABORATORIES $ 5.26
RADIOLOGY $ 2.90
ANESTHESIA $ 2.47
OPERATING ROOMS $ 5.54
SOCIAL SERVICE $ .59
MEDICAL RECORDS $ .33
DRUGS AND SUPPLIES $ 2.92
NURSING EDUCATION $ 2.26
NURSING SERVICE $11.10
PHYSICIANS' SERVICES $ 2.69
FOOD $ 4.85
LAUNDRY AND LINEN $ 1.61
DEPRECIATION $ .45
PLANT OPERATION $ 2.20
AND MAINTENANCE
ADMINISTRATION $ 1.99

1963–1964

1971–1972

national commissions to belabor the obvious. Prepayment on a capitation basis, with comprehensive services rendered by salaried groups of physicians to large consumer groups (as contrasted with *ad hoc* fee-for-service arrangements), can result in as much as a 50 percent reduction in hospitalization and surgery. Even as little as a 10 percent reduction could save $3 billion annually. With minor exceptions dictated by geographic needs, far fewer high-cost hospital facilities should be built in the U.S. Instead attention should be paid to improving existing facilities and achieving their full utilization. New construction should focus on the desperate need for more ambulatory facilities, chronic hospitals, extended-care facilities and nursing homes, so that prolonged and unnecessary use of high-cost, acute hospital facilities can be avoided. Insurance mechanisms should stress those services that have a high benefit-cost ratio. These services must include rehabilitation, family planning, health education and disease prevention.

Let me post a difficult and frustrating caveat. Death is inevitable, and as we conquer one scourge another will take its place. Medical science and technology will continue to prolong life, and the nation could expend a steadily increasing percentage of its national resources on prolonging life at any cost. Kidney dialysis, transplantation surgery, artificial heart-lung pumps—these and more to come would inevitably consume an ever increasing share of the national resources, and all attempts to reduce or hold down the costs of medical care would be doomed to failure. The heart transplant is the medical equivalent of landing men on the moon. Inevitably we must meet the question: Life for what, and at what cost? Moral, ethical and philosophical concerns must enter the decision-making process in all sectors of American life.

AVERAGE DAILY COST of hospitalization more than tripled in the eight-year period from fiscal year 1963–1964 to fiscal year 1971–1972. The amounts shown are for a single institution, the Massachusetts General Hospital, and are higher than the national average; relationships of costs, however, are probably similar in other hospitals. "Hotel costs" are shown in dark color. Routine expenses include the hotel costs as well as those items shown in medium color. Ancillary expenses (*light color*) are those for which the patient receives an itemized bill. Drugs and supplies are listed twice because some are billed to the patient separately.

X

The Medical School

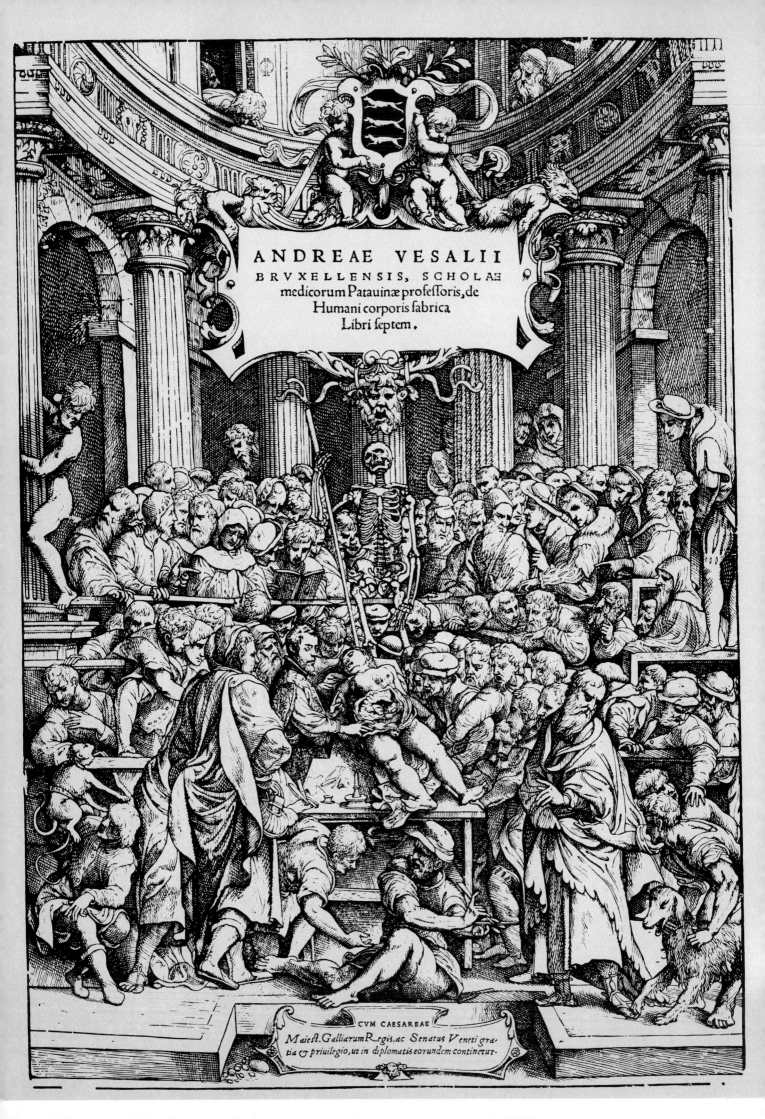

The Medical School

ROBERT H. EBERT

The training of physicians is in the midst of a period of rapid evolutionary change. The probable outcome will be the production of fewer specialists and more physicians capable of primary care

The training of physicians has passed through two periods of drastic change in America, the first in about the middle of the 18th century, when medical schools began replacing apprenticeship as the route to becoming a physician, and the second early in this century, when medical schools were for the first time put on a firm scientific basis. Today medical education is in another period of transition, which perhaps cannot be characterized as drastic but which is nonetheless substantial and significant. Among other things, it can be expected to result in a shorter period of training for physicians, an earlier exposure of medical students to patients, more opportunity for elective study and a different amalgam of specialists among the graduates.

Medical education reflects the perceived needs of both practicing physicians and the society, which utilizes medical services and pays the bills. The main link, however, is between medical schools and the profession, not only because clinical faculty members are heavily engaged in the practice of medicine but also because teaching hospitals (or medical centers, as they are now called) are a prominent component of the medical-care system and dominate one part of it. Both medical education and medical practice have evolved through a number of eras, and medical education often anticipates the transition from one era to another. In such a time there is usually tension between the

practitioner and the educator, reflecting the difference between eras, and tensions of this nature are much in evidence during the present period of change.

In the U.S. medical education and medical practice have evolved in a peculiarly American way, and it is difficult to understand the current problems of medical education without retracing that evolution. The Colonial era, which has been well described by the historian Daniel J. Boorstin, was characterized by nonprofessionalism and the involvement of lay people in medical affairs. English medicine in Colonial times was rigidly controlled by guilds and dominated by dogma. The English system was not imported to the New World, for a reason suggested in 1728 by William Byrd, a prominent official and landowner in Colonial Virginia, who said: "The New Proprietor [of New Jersey] inveigled many over by this tempting Account of the Country: that it was a Place free from those 3 great scourges of Mankind, Priests, Lawyers and Physicians. Nor did they tell a word of Lye, for the People were too poor to maintain these Learned Gentlemen." The American physician, unlike his English cousin, did everything from surgery to dispensing drugs, and he was not constrained by legal or professional regulations. Medical education was equally informal, consisting mainly of the apprentice system.

Beginning in the middle of the 18th century a number of medical depart-

ments were created in universities. The College of Philadelphia (now the University of Pennsylvania) established a professorship in the theory and practice of medicine in 1765, and similar departments were formed at King's College (now Columbia University) in 1768 and at Harvard College in 1783. It was not universities, however, but rather the proprietary medical schools (privately owned and profit-making), that dominated American medicine during nearly all of the 19th century.

The first proprietary medical school was started in Baltimore early in the 19th century. In a little more than a century 457 medical schools were founded in the U.S. and Canada, and most of them were proprietary. The proprietary schools were shockingly bad by modern standards. The only requirements for admission were the tuition and the ability to read and write. Education from the viewpoint of the students was entirely passive: the teachers lectured and the students listened. The schools had no laboratories, and frequently "chairs" of medicine and surgery were sold to the highest bidder.

It is natural to wonder how such schools could survive for so long and to ask about their relation to medical practice. Although there was much justifiable criticism of the quality of education that the schools provided, it may be that they suited the needs of the time better than the university medical schools did. Proprietary schools were a rather natural outgrowth of the informal approach to medical practice that had been established in the Colonial period, and they complemented the apprenticeship system of medical education. Moreover, they trained large numbers of physicians for the frontier, with the result that almost no small town during the 19th century was without its general practitioner. It must be remembered that there was very little in the way of a scientific base for medicine during this period and certainly little that medicine could do for a patient therapeutically, so that the physician's lack of a university education probably made little difference. Nonetheless, if one is inclined toward nostalgia for the kindly family physician of that era, one should remember that the product of the proprietary medical school was badly educated and by today's standards would be considered a menace to medical practice.

Medical education's second era of sharp transition was heralded by the Flexner report of 1910 (*Medical Education in the United States and Canada*), commissioned by the Carnegie Foundation for the Advancement of Teaching and written by Abraham Flexner, who was an educator but not a physician. Probably no report, public or private, has had a more profound effect on medical education than this one, but the Flexner report could not have been an instrument for change if it had not come at the right time. Scientific medicine had begun to flower in Europe, particularly in Germany, in the latter part of the 19th century. Histology, pathology, bacteriology and physiology became fundamental disciplines that every educated phy-

sician needed to understand in order to be more than a poorly trained technician. University medical schools were assuming a more important role by the beginning of the present century; the new medical school at Johns Hopkins University in particular was oriented toward laboratory science. Specialists were becoming increasingly powerful in the medical profession, and many of them, having obtained their training in Europe, were critical of American medical education and particularly of the proprietary school. Finally, the American Medical Association, through its Council on Medical Education and Hospitals (created in 1904), became a force for reform of medical education.

It was in this setting that Flexner made his scathing indictment of American medical education. He was a graduate of Johns Hopkins, and during a long sabbatical leave in Europe he was profoundly impressed by the German university system. After receiving his commission from the Carnegie Foundation he visited each of the 155 American medical schools then in operation.

In his report Flexner was vitriolic in his comments about proprietary medical schools. He recommended that they all be closed. As for medical schools associated with universities, he reported that they were somewhat better than the proprietary schools but still left much to

be desired. Requirements for admission were too lax and teaching was too didactic. He was particularly critical of clinical departments, expressing the view that there should be full-time clinical faculty members who were as much a part of the university as their preclinical colleagues. Only the Hopkins medical school escaped his criticism; he described it as a suitable model.

Within a remarkably short time after Flexner's report many of his recommendations were put into effect. New state licensing laws were passed that defined in considerable detail the academic requirements for admission to medical school and the subject matter to be taught there. One by one the proprietary schools closed. Medical schools were reformed. Full-time professors were recruited to head clinical departments, and clinical medicine gradually became more scientific and less pragmatic. A decade after the Flexner report medical education and medical practice in the U.S. were well launched into a new scientific era, which was to lead to the worldwide dominance of American medical education and American biomedical science.

One result of the Flexner report was a closer relationship between the medical school and the university, although the integration envisioned by Flexner was never completely achieved. In some universities the medical school was geo-

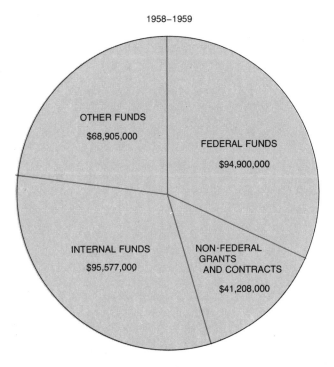
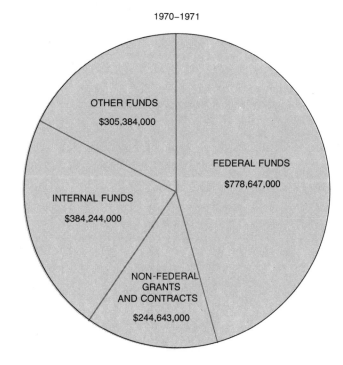

1958–1959

1970–1971

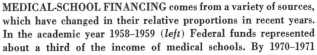

MEDICAL-SCHOOL FINANCING comes from a variety of sources, which have changed in their relative proportions in recent years. In the academic year 1958–1959 (*left*) Federal funds represented about a third of the income of medical schools. By 1970–1971 (*right*) the Federal share was about half. "Other" funds include state and local subsidies and various unrestricted gifts. The data for this chart and several others accompanying this article were assembled by *The Journal of the American Medical Association*.

graphically separate from the main university campus; in others, although the medical school was physically part of the university, the sheer size of the school's facilities and faculty made integration difficult. At best a kind of uneasy balance of power developed between medical centers and universities, and the problem remains today.

In part this problem is financial. It is not unusual for the budget of a medical school to equal or exceed the budget of the entire university less the medical school. Salaries of medical-school faculty members are characteristically higher than the faculty salaries in other departments; indeed, in some institutions the differential starts at 100 percent and goes up from there.

The problem also relates in part to issues of educational philosophy. The apprenticeship system of education has not disappeared from medicine, although the environment is totally different from the one that characterized medical training in earlier times. The medical student learns clinical medicine by caring for hospitalized patients, and he is very much a part of the hospital-ward team that consists of students, interns, residents and senior staff members. In this aspect medical education is quite different from education for the other learned professions. Law students do not deal with clients, nor do divinity students have parishes, but medical students have their own patients (for whom they share responsibility with more experienced practitioners). Medical education has one foot in the university and one foot in medical practice, and so it has never become a completely integral part of academic life.

Although many variants of the university hospital developed, and none was the precise equivalent of the German model admired by Flexner, all had certain characteristics in common. All of them had full-time clinical faculty members, at least in part; all became referral centers for patients with complex illnesses; all emphasized clinical research, and all were predominantly, if not exclusively, interested in the hospitalized patient. Over a period of time these hospitals became the centers for graduate training as well as the education of medical students. They responded admirably to the needs of the various medical specialties and developed the model programs for training the specialists.

This evolution had a profound effect on the practice of medicine, because the direct ties between academic medicine

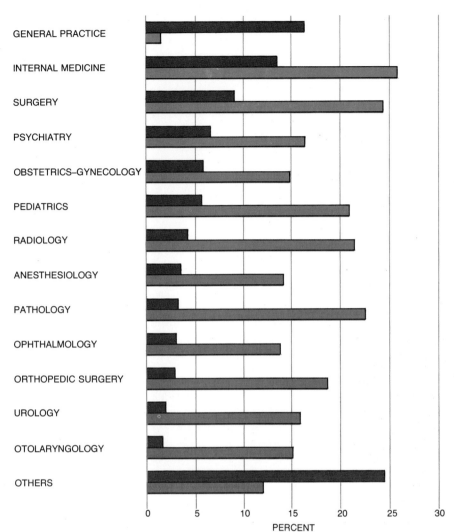

UNEVEN REPLACEMENT OF SPECIALISTS is suggested by a comparison of the percent of all physicians in each field (*gray*) with the percent of each field represented by house officers (*color*), meaning interns and residents. In other words, general practitioners are not replacing themselves, whereas most other medical specialists are being replaced in excess.

and the medical specialties hastened the deterioration of the status of the general practitioner. There were no general-practitioner models in the teaching hospital, nor did the hospital exhibit any interest in what is now called community medicine (a new term for general practice). Moreover, the products of the graduate-specialty programs who moved to community hospitals attempted to re-create there the specialty-oriented environment of the university hospital, often with considerable success.

The era of scientific medicine characterized by the changes following the Flexner report reached a culmination in the establishment (in 1937) and rapid expansion of the National Institutes of Health. Biomedical research flourished as never before in the U.S.; important advances were made in the science and technology of medicine, and university medical centers dominated not only medical education and the graduate

training of specialists but also the practice of specialty medicine. American university medical centers became the places to which affluent patients from all over the world were referred, and they also became huge research establishments. By evolving along these lines the university medical centers became increasingly detached from their local communities and their parent universities. They provided superb care for the people (rich and poor) who were fortunate enough to be hospitalized, but they assumed little or no responsibility for the communities surrounding them.

So, notwithstanding the great successes of the Flexner era, there has been a growing public dissatisfaction with medical schools and the practicing physician. Family physicians have become increasingly scarce, so that even affluent people find it difficult at times to obtain routine medical care. Medical services are poorly distributed, being concentrated heavily in the suburbs and relatively sparsely in the central city (except for the teaching hospitals) and in rural areas. As small-town general practitioners retire or die they are not replaced, and few general internists and pediatricians want to take up the solo practice of medicine in a small town. Physicians are accused of being too specialized and more interested in disease than in people.

In this context it is being argued with increasing force that medical care is a right and not a privilege and that one class of medical care should be available to everyone. Indeed, in contrast to the pressures that brought about the Flexner era, the reform of medical education and medical practice is now being pressed by forces outside medicine. They include consumer groups, members of Congress, labor, corporate industry (which pays a significant part of the health bill) and such nonmedical professionals as economists, sociologists and a variety of experts in the fields of management and public policy. The demand is for more equitable distribution of medical service, better control of cost and a change in the education of physicians.

In the turmoil of transition medical schools are being asked to do a variety of things, few of which are consistent with past missions and not all of which are consistent with one another. The schools are under pressure to increase in size, change the patterns of training for the medical specialties, enroll more women and members of minority groups, train physician assistants and more practitioners, provide clinical training for American students enrolled in foreign medical schools, experiment with the medical-care system to put more emphasis on ambulatory care and comprehensive care, provide primary care for communities adjacent to teaching hospitals and participate in regional planning. The goal of all these missions is to provide a more equitable distribution of health services. Some of the missions are directed toward increasing manpower in the health field and training new types of health professional, and other missions deal with the organization of health services. In this array of missions lies a dilemma: one cannot define with any accuracy the manpower requirements for a system of medical care that has yet to be clearly defined.

In response to social pressures and special Federal funding new medical schools have been established and existing schools have increased in size. Five new schools opened in the fall of 1971, bringing the total in the U.S. to 108. The 108 schools enrolled 43,650 students in the academic year 1971–1972, which was an increase of 3,163 students over the previous year. Between 1947–1948 and 1967–1968 first-year enrollment rose from 6,487 to 9,479, which was an increase of 2,992; then in the next five years it rose by 2,882, or almost as much as in the preceding 20 years. Such other groups as interns, residents and paramedical people, which are also part of the teaching responsibility of medical-school faculties, likewise increased in size.

For the academic year 1971–1972 the 12,361 first-year places in medical schools had 29,172 applicants. The ratio of 2.4 applicants per acceptance was the highest since 1951–1952, which marked the end of the postwar pressure for admission to medical schools. Of the applicants accepted in 1971, 24 percent had an undergraduate academic average of A; only 6 percent had a C average. (In 1961 12.2 percent of the applicants accepted had an A average and 17.4 percent had C.) The 1971 group included 13.6 percent who were women and 7

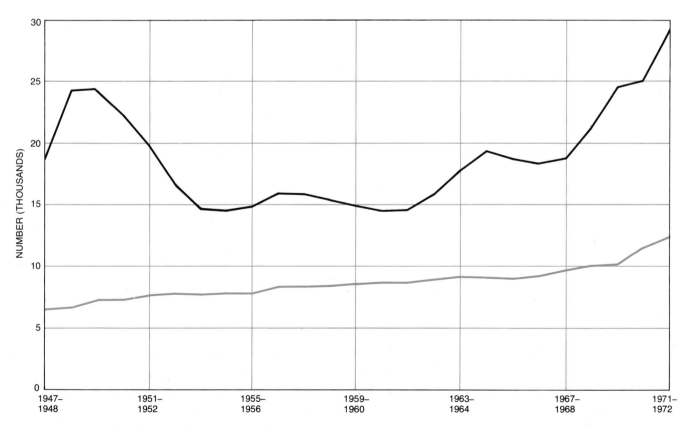

PRESSURE ON MEDICAL SCHOOLS appears in a comparison of the number of applicants (*black*) with the number of acceptances (*color*) for the period beginning with the academic year 1947–1948 and continuing through the class that entered medical school in 1971. Pressure for admission is also reflected by the fact that the number of applications made by each individual has risen from an average of three in 1947 to 7.2 in 1971. The ratio of applicants to acceptances was 3.5 in 1948, fell to 1.7 in 1960 and rose to 2.4 in 1971.

percent who were members of minority groups. Judging from the overall attrition rate of 1.34 percent in 1971–1972, it could be expected that nearly all the students who entered medical school in 1971 would finish medical school and complete further training.

Since statistics are lifeless, one wonders about what kind of people the new medical students are. They are a mixed group, probably less homogeneous than earlier classes, but they have one thing in common: they have been successful both academically and socially. They have succeeded in part because they have been competitive, and yet many of them are weary of the competition, even though they will have to compete again for internships and residencies. In general they are serious-minded, and many of them are concerned about social issues, including the lack of equity in the medical-care system. They want to make a good living, but few of them aspire to wealth.

What happens to the applicants who are rejected? Some of them reapply or seek careers related to medicine. A significant number enter foreign medical schools. In 1970–1971 the number of American students enrolled in foreign medical schools was 3,922. More than half of them were at the Autonomous University of Guadalajara in Mexico and the University of Bologna. The medical education they receive is inferior, and they are looked on as part of the pool of foreign medical graduates.

Even with the increasing enrollment in American medical schools, medicine in the U.S. draws heavily on the pool of foreign medical graduates. The expanding role of the hospitals, which includes being in effect the family physician to the poor, means that more internships and residencies are offered than can be filled by graduates of American medical schools. Many of these places (18,436 of the 54,359 house officers on duty in American hospitals in 1971) are filled by foreign medical graduates, a considerable number of whom are from Asia.

House officers represent a significant proportion (15.3 percent) of the pool of practicing physicians. It is noteworthy that at the end of 1971 only 1.4 percent of the house officers were taking their training in general-practice programs, although 16.3 percent of all physicians in the U.S. are general practitioners. What is perhaps more important is the distribution of interns and residents between programs oriented toward primary care (general practice, internal medicine, pediatrics and obstetrics and gynecology) and programs oriented toward other specialties. Only 37 percent of the interns and residents are in the specialties related to primary care, and not all of them will be concerned with primary care when they finish training. Yet from 55 to 60 percent of the physicians in comprehensive-care programs, such as prepaid group practice, are recruited from the primary-care specialties.

The fact is that the medical schools do not know how many specialists of one type or another are needed. The health-maintenance organizations, such as the Kaiser-Permanente program, can provide an indication on the basis of their experience in dealing with large populations. They have found specialists such as surgeons to be in oversupply and physicians in such fields as internal medicine and pediatrics to be in short supply. In other words, the output of the medical schools has been geared more to the perceived needs of the profession than to the apparent needs of the society.

Medical schools are also responsible for training the growing numbers of physician assistants, who are conceived of as professionals who can increase the productivity of physicians and provide some of the primary care in areas of need. They would have a basic medical education but would not receive the M.D. degree. By last November the number of programs of this type that had been approved by the Council on Medical Education of the American Medical Association was 17, and 15 others had applied for accreditation. As yet there is no uniformity of training for these professionals and no clear conception of the role or roles they will fill.

The number of people teaching full time in medical schools has grown at an even greater rate than the student bodies. Moreover, the full-time faculty of more than 29,000 is supplemented by a part-time faculty of almost 58,000. (Medical-school teaching is faculty-intensive because so much of it involves small groups of from two to four students.) Most clinical faculty members are specialists and many of the full-time clinical faculty members are subspecialists. Few of them are interested in problems of primary care—a fact reflected by the large enrollments in the residency programs in the medical specialties.

The question of the financing of medical education is too complex to be treated in any detail here, but several points

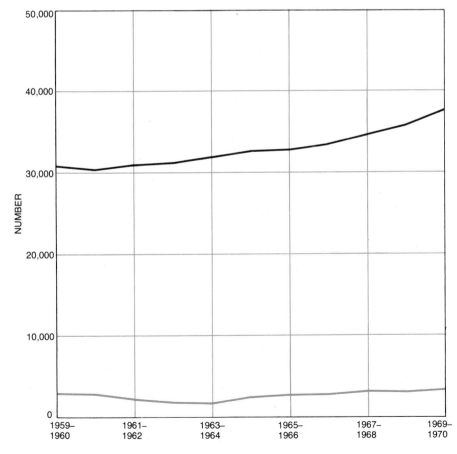

FOREIGN MEDICAL SCHOOLS are educating increasing numbers of Americans, reflecting the difficulty many applicants have getting into medical schools in the U.S. Chart compares number of students in U.S. medical schools (*black*) with number of U.S. students in foreign medical schools (*color*), according to data from Institute of International Education.

merit emphasis. First, the financing comes from many sources [*see illustration on page 104*]. Second, the cost is increasing (from $319 million in 1958–1959 to $1.7 billion in 1970–1971). Third, one is dealing here with joint costs of teaching (a cost complicated by the fact that the students range from newly admitted college graduates to senior residents), patient care and research—and even industry has yet to find a satisfactory way of unambiguously attributing joint costs to the production of different products. Fourth, the source of funding influences the direction of medical-school activity. For example, Federal funding from 1950 to 1968 came largely from the National Institutes of Health, and during this period full-time faculty increased 422 percent, graduate and postdoctoral students 208 percent, university-hospital interns and residents 280 percent and medical students 42 percent. These patterns are changing with a change in the pattern of Federal funding. Fifth, a high proportion of medical students receive support from scholarships and loans, and the amounts are increasing. (It is worthy of note that the U.S. is the only major country that ex-

pects the student or his family to pay for a medical education.)

The trends in financing have been reflected in the design of the medical-school curriculum. Two fundamental changes in curriculum have been pioneered by Case Western Reserve School of Medicine, namely early involvement with patients and integrated teaching. The traditional medical-school curriculum separated the first two years of preclinical teaching from the last two clinical years, and teaching was departmental. Many schools now introduce the student to the care of patients much earlier and subscribe to the joint teaching of pathophysiology by both basic scientists and clinicians. In addition more time is elective (often as much as one and a half years), allowing the development of "tracks" through medical school whereby the student can emphasize the biomedical sciences or the social and behavioral sciences.

More striking changes are likely to materialize, because it is becoming increasingly difficult to define the limits of medical education. The biological sciences (including biochemistry, microbiology and cell biology) were once re-

garded as the exclusive domain of medical schools but are now increasingly taught to undergraduates. At the other end of the spectrum, medical faculties are increasingly involved in the education of house officers.

In addition concern is growing over the length of the educational process, particularly in the light of the growing debt load of students. Is it realistic to require four years of college, four years of medical school and from three to seven years of postdoctoral training? Is it even good pedagogy? The process could be telescoped by shortening college to two or three years, shortening medical schools (a number of them give the M.D. degree after three years, although the time is saved mainly by eliminating vacations) and cutting down the period of internship and residency. Time could also be saved by various combinations of the student's clinical work in medical school and his period of work as a house officer.

Two final comments should be made about the medical-school environment. First, the hospitalized patient has been the principal focus of clinical teaching, for good reasons, namely that it is easier for the medical student to share responsibility for the hospitalized patient than for the outpatient and that with the hospitalized patient the student can work at a slower pace. It is becoming increasingly evident, however, that a better structure is needed for ambulatory care so that both medical students and house officers can gain more experience with such patients. Second, it has been argued that since physicians, nurses, physician assistants and social workers must function as a team, they should be educated together. It seems unlikely that they will be, however, because of the different levels of scientific competence required for the different disciplines.

As for the future of medical education, accurate prediction is impossible because of the influences that will be brought to bear by a variety of events that have yet to come and decisions that have yet to be made. The evolution of the nation's system of medical care will be a predominant factor. When national health insurance comes, as it will, will it preserve the fee-for-service system or will it encourage prepayment for all care? Will care be provided by large groups of medical professionals, and will hospitals continue to dominate the system? The method of financing medical education in the future will also be a factor, particularly if direct support of medical schools by tax dollars on a per capita

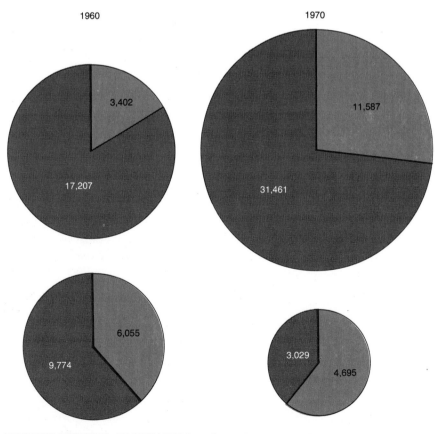

1960

3,402

17,207

1970

11,587

31,461

6,055

9,774

3,029

4,695

FOREIGN MEDICAL GRADUATES have been playing an important role in U.S. medicine, as reflected by the number of them on duty as house officers in American hospitals. In 1960, in hospitals affiliated with medical schools (*top*), 17,207 house officers (*gray*) were graduates of American medical schools and 3,402 (*color*) were foreign medical graduates. The proportion of foreign medical graduates in hospitals not affiliated with medical schools (*bottom*) was higher. In 1970 both types of hospital had more foreign medical graduates.

basis is expanded. For example, a recent act of Congress authorizing capitation allowances to medical schools required expansion of enrollment as a condition of support.

Public attitudes will be important. If medical services continue to be in short supply at the same time that large numbers of qualified applicants cannot gain admission to medical school, the pressure to increase the size and number of the medical schools will be substantial. Moreover, both Congress and the executive branch of the Federal Government are likely in such a case to take the position that medical education is too expensive for what it produces.

The attitudes of students may also be a factor in the future of medical education. How much debt will a student be willing to shoulder if physicians become salaried? How much will the student insist on "relevance" in the curriculum at the expense of basic medical sciences?

Having entered these disclaimers, I shall venture a few predictions. First, the total educational experience will be shortened so that much of what is now taught in the first year and a half of medical school will be presented at the undergraduate level. In addition there will be a fusing of clinical training at the medical-student level with internship and residency, so that the total amount of time spent in giving the student clinical experience will be shortened.

Second, the character of medical schools will be altered. The basic medical sciences will become an integral part of the university, whereas clinical training will become even more detached from the university, although it will remain under the university umbrella.

Third, physician assistants will not replace physicians as providers of primary care except in remote rural areas, and even there the assistants will have circumscribed tasks and ready access to direction from physicians. Fourth, the number of medical students receiving the M.D. degree will rise, perhaps even to the point of oversupply if care is better organized. This development would cut down or eliminate the importation of foreign medical graduates. Fifth, the number and quality of residency programs will be brought under tighter regulation, and training opportunities for primary-care physicians will gain predominance over programs for specialists. Finally, the number of women and members of minority groups entering medicine will increase, thereby aiding in the solution of the problem of equitably distributing medical services.

XI

The Medical Economy

The Medical Economy

MARTIN S. FELDSTEIN

Over 95 percent of the American people have some form of health insurance, but the coverage is shallow and is responsible for much of the 500 percent rise in the cost of hospital care since 1950

Inflation of costs and inequity of distribution are the central issues in the public debate about American health care today. The nature and significance of these problems have generally been misunderstood. Cost inflation is important because it reflects the serious misallocation of resources and the failure of the health-care system to reflect individual preferences. Moreover, for some families high medical costs create financial hardship and present a barrier to adequate medical care.

There is a peculiar economic characteristic of medical care that is largely responsible for its current problems. It is necessary to examine this characteristic first if we are to understand the problems of medical care and to evaluate the proposals for its reform. Although there are many ways in which medical care differs from the other goods and services households buy, one feature dominates all others. For most types of goods and services a family can reasonably predict its annual expenditure. In contrast, spending on medical care is very uncertain. The nature of this uncertainty is particularly significant.

The distribution of the annual expenditure on health care among families is extremely skewed. Whereas most families spend relatively little on health care, a few families are obliged to spend a great deal. A study of health spending by Federal Government employees in 1969 showed that slightly more than half of the families with two adults and two children spent less than $260 but that 10 percent of the families spent more than $1,500 and 5 percent spent more than $2,600. These annual amounts include both the families' direct out-of-pocket expenditures and payments by insurance companies.

The inherent uncertainty of family medical-care costs creates a demand for health insurance. By paying a fixed annual premium the family lowers the risk of a much higher unpredictable expense. Since insurance companies pool many families, they can sell insurance at a premium that is little more than the mean (or actuarial) value of the insured risk. For example, the mean cost of health expenses in the study of Government employees just cited is about $610. If complete insurance were available (that is, insurance with no deductibles, no coinsurance and no limits to benefits), the family could avoid all risk of serious financial hardship by paying only slightly more than $610.

The incentive to insure becomes stronger as the risk of a very large expenditure increases and as the distribution of expenses becomes more skewed. Thus insurance coverage is most complete for hospital care: in 1972 private insurance paid about 80 percent of consumers' expenditure for such care, leaving only 20 percent to be paid out of pocket. Although insurance pays nearly half of consumers' expenditures for physicians' services, this reflects the fact that the coverage for large surgical fees is much more complete than it is for ambulatory care by specialists and general practitioners.

Federal tax policy encourages the use of insurance by a subsidy that now exceeds $3 billion per year. Individuals can deduct from their income a substantial fraction (usually about half) of the premiums they pay for health insurance. More important, employer payments for health insurance are excluded from the taxable income of both the employee and the employer. These premiums are also not subject to the 10.4 percent social-security payroll tax or to state income taxes. Even for a relatively low income

family the inducement to buy insurance can be substantial. Because of the income and payroll taxes a married man with two children who now earns $8,000 a year will take home only $70 for every $100 his employer adds to his salary. If his employer buys health insurance for him instead, the full $100 can be applied against the premium. In this case a dollar buys nearly 50 percent more health-care services if it is paid through an insurance premium than if it is received in wages and used to buy services directly. For workers in higher tax brackets the incentive is even stronger. In the aggregate the Government subsidy exceeds the total administrative costs and profits of the health-insurance industry. The special tax policy has no doubt contributed significantly to the nearly twentyfold increase in non-Government insurance benefits since 1950 and to the concurrent tripling of the fraction of consumer health expenditures paid by insurance [*see top illustration on next page*].

In addition to providing protection against unpredictable medical expenses, health insurance substantially lowers the net price of care that the patient faces when he consumes health services. There is now substantial evidence that such changes in the net price of care affect how much the patient uses the services available. The growth of insurance coverage has therefore been a mixed blessing. Because hospital care is more completely insured than other health services, insurance distorts the pattern of health care toward the use of expensive hospital inpatient care even when less expensive ambulatory care would be equally efficient. Moreover, because surgical services and other specialists' care are more completely in-

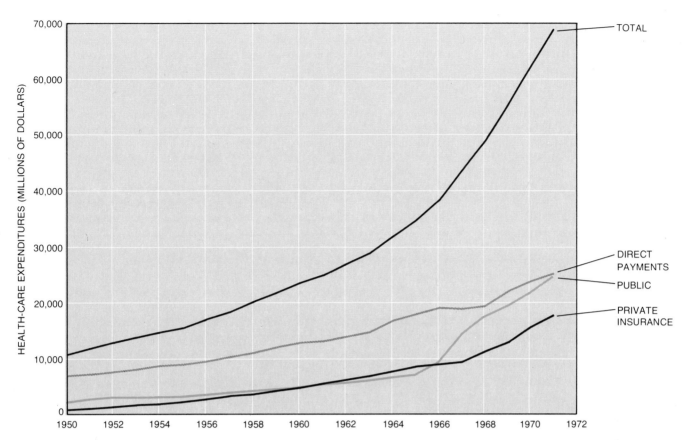

PAYMENTS FOR HEALTH CARE come from three main sources: from public funds, from private insurance benefits and in the form of direct payments by the consumer. Between 1950 and 1971 public expenditures for health increased tenfold (to $24.9 billion), private insurance benefits increased eighteenfold (to $17.9 billion) and direct payments about three-and-a-half-fold (to $25.2 billion).

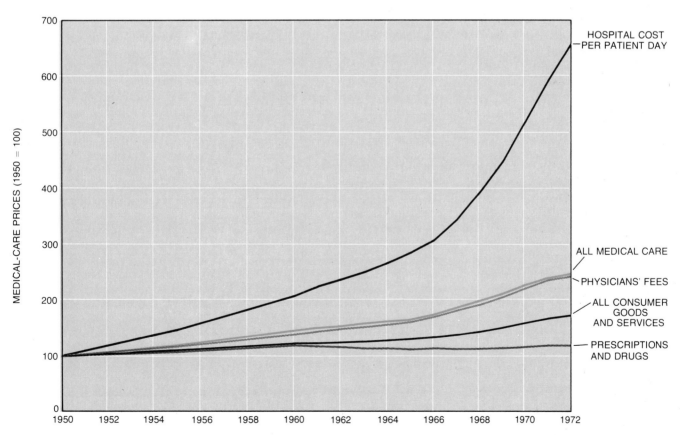

COST OF HOSPITAL CARE has risen dramatically since 1950, far outstripping the rise in physicians' fees. As a result the overall cost of medical care has gone up faster than the average of all goods and services in the consumer price index. The indexes are adjusted to make 1950 equal to 100. Prescriptions and drugs have risen the least of all health-care costs: from 100 to 119. The cost of over-the-counter drugs actually fell in the years between 1950 and 1972, but the drop was more than offset by the doubling of prescription costs.

sured than care by general practitioners is, insurance distorts the use of physicians' services. (The more heavily insured specialties are also able to charge higher fees, which in turn attracts more physicians into those fields.) More generally, because insured patients pay only a small fraction of the extra cost of more expensive care, insurance distorts all aspects of patient care toward the increased use of services and toward the use of more expensive services. In short, health insurance not only pays for medical expenses but also shapes the volume and form of medical spending.

The fact that health insurance increases the family's expected expenditure on medical care has three important implications. First, as insurance becomes more complete a point is reached where any additional care that might be consumed does not seem worth the greater total premiums and out-of-pocket spending. Families will therefore prefer to be less than fully insured. In the absence of complete insurance families are left exposed to the risk of high out-of-pocket expenses. Second, the process of balancing a reduction of risk against the added cost of extra services implies that the more risky types of expenditure will be more fully insured. This leads to the buying of more complete insurance for hospital bills and surgical fees and therefore distorts the mix of services that are used. Finally, the sensitivity of healthcare demand to the extent of insurance coverage has been a major cause of the inflation of health costs.

Over the past two decades medicalcare costs have risen more rapidly than any other component of the consumer price index. Whereas the total index rose 74 percent from 1950 to 1972, the medical-care component rose 145 percent. The increase in the average cost per patient-day in community hospitals was more dramatic: from $16 in 1950 to $103 in 1972, a rise of more than 500 percent. In contrast, physicians' fees increased at the same average rate as all services (excluding rent) in the consumer price index [*see bottom illustration on page 113*]. It is useful, therefore, to concentrate attention on the inflation of hospital costs.

Perhaps the most frequently heard explanation for the explosion of hospital costs is that hospitals are technologically and managerially inefficient; they get less output for their input than ordinary business firms. But even if there are reasons to criticize the current level of hospital production efficiency, there is no

reason to believe that the efficiency of hospital management has actually been rapidly declining. Inefficiency could not possibly account for an increase of more than 500 percent in 22 years in the cost per patient-day. If hospitals are less efficient than other institutions in using inputs to produce services, hospital costs will be higher than they should be but they will not be rising faster.

Rising labor costs are also often cited as the primary cause of hospital-cost inflation. It is true that wages and salaries constitute a large share of hospital costs and that hospital wage rates have risen more rapidly than the general level of wages in the economy has. Nevertheless, this does not adequately account for the inflation of hospital costs. From 1955 through 1971 labor costs per patient-day rose 270 percent. As a fraction of the total bill, however, labor costs remained nearly constant at about 60 percent. Thus nonlabor costs have risen about as fast as labor costs. Moreover, about a fifth of the increase in labor costs reflected a rise in the number of personnel per day. Only 34 percent of the increase in total cost per patient-day can be accounted for by higher wages per se. Since hospital wage rates rose 160 percent while general industrial wages rose 103 percent, the excess hospital wage increase actually accounts for very little of the unusually rapid rise in hospital costs.

It is nevertheless interesting to ask why hospital wages have risen more rapidly than wages in general. A frequent assertion is that hospital wages are "catching up," implying that they were significantly below the wages in industry generally and are now coming closer. This is correct as a description but misleading as an explanation. In order to assess the catching-up argument it is useful to distinguish between occupations in which hospitals hire only a small fraction of workers (for example clerical and maintenance workers) from an occupation such as nursing, which is essentially confined to the hospital industry. There is no reason why the average wage for all hospital personnel should be equal to or close to the average wage in manufacturing. Although there is a general tendency for wages in any occupation to become equal in all industries, substantial differences can persist for a long time. The expression "catching up" implies that after hospital wages had caught up they would increase at about the same rate as wages in other industries. There are, however, many examples of occupations in which

hospitals have recently begun paying higher wages than other industries in the same geographic area. Unless we understand why hospital wages have been going up we cannot predict how they will behave in the future.

Unionization and the minimum-wage law are often cited as causes of rising hospital wages. It is difficult to establish exactly how important either factor has been. It has been estimated that the changes in the Federal minimum-wage law have caused hospital cost per patient-day to rise about $2, hardly a significant amount. Although the unionization of hospitals has been advancing, it still accounts for only a small fraction of personnel and an even smaller fraction of hospitals. Clearly neither of these two factors is primarily responsible for the increase in hospital wages.

Part of the wage rise is no doubt due to the hospitals' increased demand for personnel. My own feeling is that hospital wages have also gone up as hospitals have become better able to absorb the added costs and therefore have become more willing to accede to the pressure for higher wages. In some instances hospitals have actually encouraged those who demand higher wages, knowing that the money to meet the increased cost would be available from private insurance, Medicare and Medicaid. The best example of this is the rise in interns' salaries from token payments of a few hundred dollars a year in the 1950's to more than $10,000 today.

Hospital-cost inflation has also been attributed to a low rate of technical progress. I think that is clearly and obviously false. Hospitals have been the scene of extremely rapid changes in technology, but the character of these changes has been different from that in other industries. It has not been costreducing. Technical progress in hospitals has not involved making the old products more cheaply but rather making a new product or a new range of products.

Why have hospitals moved toward increasingly expensive ways of doing new things rather than in the direction of providing old products more cheaply and efficiently? Although some of this undoubtedly reflects the path of basic scientific progress, it is our method of financing health services and its impact on demand that primarily determine the general pattern of technical progress that has developed.

The final and most important explanation for rising hospital costs is the rapid increase in demand. The steady increase in family income and in levels of education and, more significant, the expansion of health-care insurance have led to a rapid growth in the demand for sophisticated hospital services. This growth of demand should not be misunderstood. It is partly an increase in the desired number of hospital admissions and in the average duration of stay per case. It is also, however, that people are willing to pay a higher price for the same level of service and are eager to obtain more expensive medical and hospital care.

The usual economic analysis implies that prices rise because supply does not increase as rapidly as demand. In the case of hospitals it is precisely because supply has kept pace with demand that hospital costs have gone up. Hospitals have responded to the increasing demand and the increased willingness to pay for sophisticated services by providing those services.

The growth of insurance has played the dominant role in increasing the demand. In 1950 insurance paid only 37 percent of consumers' expenditures for hospital care; the balance was paid out of pocket. Since the average cost per patient-day was then $16, the out-of-pocket expenditure came to $10. In 1972 the average cost per patient-day was $103, of which insurance paid 82 percent, or $84.50. The net out-of-pocket cost to the patient was therefore only $18.50. Even the small increase from $10 to $18.50 overstates the real rise in the net cost of a day of hospital care. Because of the general rise in consumer prices, $18.50 in 1972 could buy only as much as $10.65 could buy in 1950 [*see the illustration on page 116*]. In real terms the net cost to the patient of hospital care has hardly changed in 20 years. It is not surprising, therefore, that consumer demand has encouraged and supported the rapid growth of advanced and expensive hospital services.

The emphasis I have put on the changing nature of the hospital product raises an awkward question. Implicit in every discussion of the inflation of hospital costs is the assumption that the rise in cost per patient-day has been excessive and should not continue at the same rate in the future. But if this rise primarily reflects a changing product rather than either increasing inefficiency or a low rate of technical progress, in what sense are rising hospital costs really a problem? The answer in brief is that the current type of costly medical care does not correspond to what consumers (and their physicians too) would regard as

being appropriate if their choices were not distorted by insurance.

The effect of prepaying health care through insurance, both private and government, is to encourage hospitals to provide a more expensive product than the consumers actually wish to purchase. Although the consumer pays for more expensive care through higher insurance premiums, at the time of illness the insured patient's demand for care reflects the net price, that is, the hospital's charge net of the insurance benefits. Because this net out-of-pocket cost appears so modest, the patient is willing to buy more expensive care than he would if he were not insured. It is important to recognize that the increased

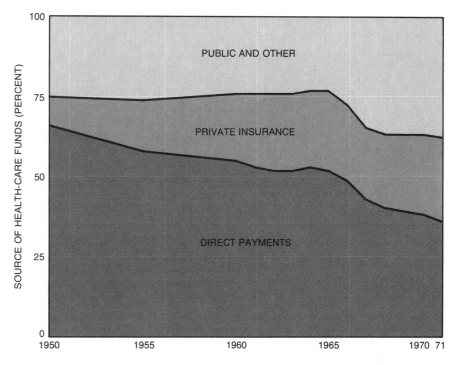

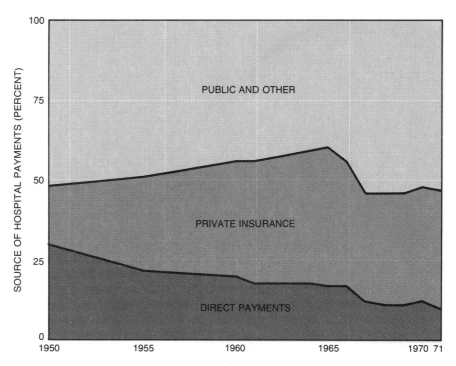

STEADY DROP IN OUT-OF-POCKET, OR DIRECT, PAYMENTS has been the outstanding feature of the way American families met their medical bills. Whereas two-thirds of all health-care expenditures were paid out of pocket in 1950, only a little more than a third are paid that way today (*top*). For hospital-care costs the fraction paid directly by the consumer was lower to begin with and has dropped even faster: from 30 percent to 10 (*bottom*).

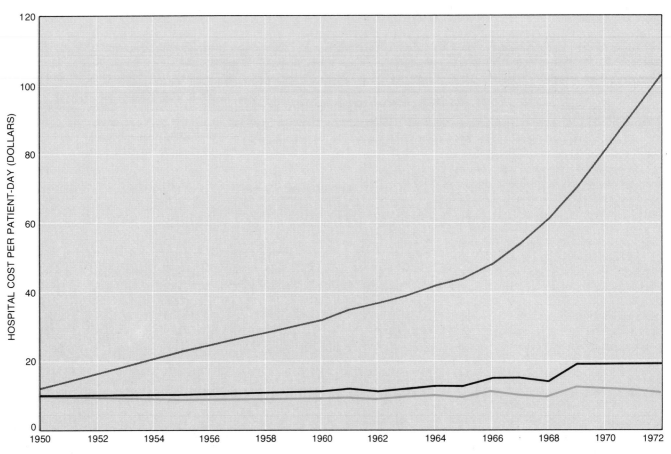

NET COST OF HOSPITAL CARE in constant dollars (*curve in solid color*) has scarcely risen since 1950, although the average cost per patient-day in community hospitals has soared from $16 to $103 (*gray curve*). In current dollars the out-of-pocket cost for patient-day has risen from $10 to $19 (*black curve*). Whereas private insurance paid $6 of a day's hospital cost in 1950, it paid $84 in 1972.

demand reflects the lower net price associated with insurance and not just the fact that without insurance it would be hard for some families to obtain money to pay for expensive care. Insurance can increase the demand for expensive care as much among affluent families with substantial assets as among families with lower incomes and small savings.

Unfortunately the production of high-cost hospital care is a self-reinforcing process: the risk of very expensive hospital care stimulates patients to prepay hospital bills through relatively comprehensive insurance, while the growth of such insurance tends to make hospital care more expensive. In this way our current method of financing hospital care denies consumers the opportunity to register effectively their preferences between higher-cost and lower-cost hospital care.

Today more than 95 percent of the population are covered by some form of health insurance. Since the introduction of Medicare and Medicaid in 1966 the aged and the poor generally have had more complete coverage than the non-aged and the non-poor. The major inequities that remain are due to the typical form of health insurance and the characteristic uncertainty associated with medical expenses.

Although insurance in the aggregate pays a substantial fraction of medical bills and an even greater share of hospital expenses, individual coverage varies widely. Low-paid workers, individuals who are frequently jobless and those who are self-employed or who work in small firms are likely to have little insurance. They and their families must pay a large part of their medical bills directly out of pocket. Moreover, because the growth of insurance has raised the price of medical care these bills are larger than they would be otherwise.

Families that are not insured through employer groups can buy coverage only on very disadvantageous terms. Insurance companies know that people who are most likely to buy individual policies generally expect higher-than-average medical expenses. When the companies raise their premiums to reflect this self-selection, some of the healthier families decide not to buy insurance or to buy less than they would otherwise. The fundamental asymmetry of information between the patient and the insurer leads to a very high premium for self-selecting insurees and a resulting underinsurance of that segment of the population.

For most families insurance coverage is generally quite "shallow." The typical policy pays a high fraction of small and moderate bills but imposes a variety of ceilings on use and an effective overall ceiling on benefits. Thus families incurring large medical bills often find that their insurance pays only a small fraction. A 1963 survey by the National Opinion Research Center found that the mean annual expenditure for medical care among the families surveyed was $370, and that about a fifth of the families had expenses in excess of $500. Among the insured families that spent more than $500 only a third received benefits exceeding half of their expenditure, and another third received benefits of less than a fifth of their expenditure. In spite of the growth of major medical insurance since 1963 health insurance today still fails to provide most families with protection against very large expenses.

The absence of deep coverage leaves a significant residue of financial hardship and discourages people from seeking care because of its potential expense. That families with an income below average (but still above the poverty level) are most likely to be uninsured or to have very shallow coverage aggravates the inequity of the random dispersion of large medical expenses. In addition, whereas an out-of-pocket expenditure of $500 might pose little hardship for a family with an income of $10,000 and some savings, the same expense would be a severe burden for a low-income family. Much of the financial inequity of our current system occurs because insurance has concentrated on providing a method of prepaying small and moderate bills instead of covering the large expenses that impose a financial burden. To prevent such financial hardship insurance coverage would have to be more complete for lower-income families than for higher-income ones.

Contrary to a widespread impression low-income families do not receive less medical care than the rest of the population. Even in the period before Medicaid (the program of Federal and state governments for financing health care for low-income families) the evidence indicates that the poor got as much hospital care as people with higher incomes. A Government survey for 1963–1964 showed an age-adjusted hospital-admission rate of 124 admissions per 1,000 people in families with an annual income of less than $2,000, 142 admissions per 1,000 in families with an income between $2,000 and $4,000 and only 120 admissions per 1,000 in families with an income of more than $10,000. Members of families in the highest income group also stayed in the hospital for fewer days per episode, on the average, than patients of lower income. The quality of care received by the higher-income families may have been better, but firm evidence is lacking. Members of high-income families may also have better health and therefore less reason to seek hospital care; again there is no adequate evidence.

The use of physicians' services now shows almost no relation to income. A 1970 national survey for the Department of Health, Education, and Welfare showed that 68 percent of people aged 18 to 64 in low-income families saw a physician during the survey year; for middle- and high-income families the fractions were 69 and 70 percent. Moreover, mean visits per person were highest in the low-income group [*see illustration on page 118*].

The survey also contradicts the common assertion that physicians' services are unavailable to low-income residents of central cities. Seventy-one percent of the people between 18 and 64 in low-income families living in central cities saw a physician in the survey year, slightly more than the 69 percent for the total survey population in that age group [*see illustration on this page*]. Although physician visits in the central city by low-income children and the low-income aged were less frequent than they were in high-income families, it is clear that this reflects household demand rather than a lack of physicians in central cities.

The evidence thus suggests that the

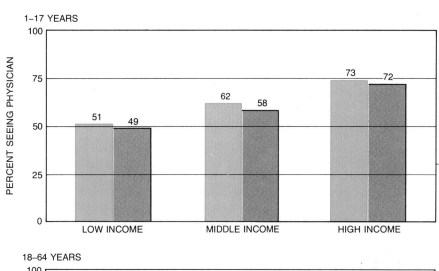

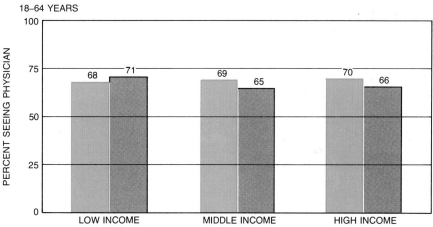

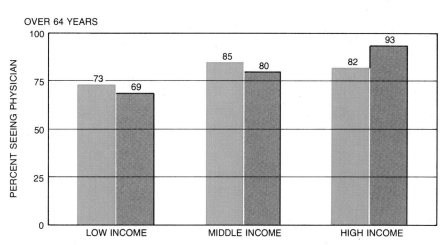

MORE THAN HALF OF ALL AMERICANS SEE A PHYSICIAN at least once a year, except for the children of low-income families who live in the central city. Even in that age group 49 percent see a physician once a year (*gray bar at extreme upper left*). The bars in color represent all individuals; the gray bars represent central-city residents. More of the high-income elderly in the central city visit doctors than members of any other group do.

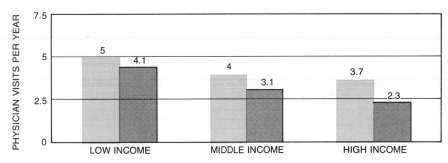

MEAN NUMBER OF PHYSICIAN VISITS PER YEAR decreases steadily with increasing family income. Bars in color represent visits by whites, bars in gray visits by nonwhites. The mean number of physician visits per year for all whites is 4.1 visits, for nonwhites 3.6.

differences among income groups in the use of health care are relatively unimportant. The significant inequities are of two types. First, all families may suffer substantial financial hardship if they incur medical expenses that are large with respect to their income. Second, some families are prevented by their form of employment from buying adequate insurance at a fair premium and are therefore much more likely to face large out-of-pocket costs or to be deterred from seeking needed medical care. Although the deprivation of care may be very small in relation to the total services provided, the consequences can obviously be quite serious.

The general increase in the cost of health care and in the personal risk of serious financial hardship has created substantial pressure for changes in the financing and organization of health services. Some form of a national health-insurance program is the most common proposal. For those who currently have little or no insurance such a Government program would be of great value. For most of the population, however, it might do no more than substitute the financing of insurance premiums through the tax system for the current voluntary employer-employee purchase of insurance. Moreover, such a substantial increase in taxes could significantly distort the supply of work effort and give rise to the inefficient use of resources in the economy as a whole.

Unless the structure of the national health-insurance coverage were very different from the typical policies of today, national health insurance would not remove the risk of financial hardship and would aggravate the problem of cost inflation. To prevent financial hardship and the undesirable deprivation of needed care the insurance coverage should limit the family's maximum medical expenditure to a reasonable fraction of family income. To avoid the continuing

inflation of hospital costs the insurance should concentrate on preventing large out-of-pocket expenses instead of prepaying a substantial proportion of typical hospital bills.

In contrast, if everyone in the population had the very comprehensive insurance of the type provided by Medicare, hospital inflation would no longer be checked by limits in patients' willingness to pay for more expensive care. The level and growth of hospital costs would have to be determined by some type of regulatory agency. The experiences of Canada and of several European countries indicate that governments have generally been unsuccessful in holding down hospital costs even when in principle they have the authority to do so. Moreover, even if the government could set the level of hospital costs, this would make the nature and quality of hospital care completely insensitive to consumer preferences.

Preserving and improving the responsiveness of health care to the preferences of the patients is likely to be the most difficult task in our future health-care system. Until now the development of our health services has been guided by the demands of individual patients and their physicians. The dramatic changes in medical practice and the growing sophistication in hospital care during the past 50 years have reflected the individually expressed willingness to pay for better medical care. As we have seen, however, the demand signals to which the health system responds have become increasingly distorted in favor of high-cost institutional care by the growth of insurance.

The inability of our current system to accurately reflect the public's preferences about the level of medical spending has induced demands for a greater use of detailed controls and regulations. These could be superimposed on our current system of financing or made an integral part of a comprehensive national

health-care plan. The case for such controls has often been supported by a false analogy to regulated industries or to planning in fields such as transportation. In the health sector there would be neither the usual problem of controlling profit rates nor the market information about consumers' preferences that characterizes planning and regulation in other sectors. In contrast, the basic difficulty of health-sector planning is that with comprehensive insurance the responsible authorities cannot possibly have the information required to provide reasoned answers to the most important questions. More specifically, planners must decide such things as the average hospital cost per patient-day, the number of patient-days per capita and ultimately the share of national income that is devoted to health care. In the short run little harm would result from merely maintaining current standards or a low rate of increase. But how would the long-run evolution of the health sector be guided?

Setting the quantity and quality of health services involves balancing health care against other forms of consumption that compete for the same national resources. An appropriate allocation of resources must therefore reflect consumer preferences. Neither medical science nor economic analysis can provide an adequate guide. Relying on the political budgeting process would only make spending for health care as arbitrary as the current national outlay for defense and scientific research. No amount of consumer representation in the planning process could ever provide an accurate measure of consumer preferences if the financing of care is separated from this planning process. The more centralized the control is and the greater the reliance on general-revenue Government funds is, the more difficult it would be to register consumers' preferences.

We should not lose sight of the way in which our health-care system might instead be reformed. It is important that we develop an approach that is appropriate to the advanced technology of today's medical care and the ever increasing affluence of the American people. Too much of the current debate relies on ideas about the delivery of medical care that have been inherited from a period with quite different technological and economic conditions. The challenge to public policy is to find new methods of organization and financing that protect families from the risk of financial hardship while making the future development of health care more responsive to the preferences of the people.

XII

The Medical Business

The Medical Business

JAMES L. GODDARD

U.S. sales of drugs, medical supplies and medical equipment are $11 billion per year. The Food and Drug Administration closely supervises the drugs but has little authority over the other items

The biggest item in the average American's budget after food, shelter, clothing and transportation is medical care. It is also the fastest-rising major component. Between 1950 and 1972, while the four leading items were increasing about 200 percent, the cost of medical care was increasing more than 400 percent. In 1950 medical care absorbed only 4.6 percent of the average budget; 22 years later it accounted for 7.5 percent. The nation's total health bill in 1972 was $70 billion, or $350 per capita. In this article I shall be concerned with the substantial fraction of the total medical-care bill that supports the "medical business": the $11 billion expended for drugs, medical supplies and equipment. To put the $11 billion in perspective, it is roughly a third of what Americans spent in 1972 on new automobiles.

In the field of ethical pharmaceuticals —drugs sold only on prescription—there are some 22,000 trade-name products in the marketplace. In the field of devices, medical equipment and supplies there is no reliable estimate of the number of products manufactured but it almost certainly exceeds 20,000. They range from cotton balls, sutures and tongue depressors to $100,000 blood-analysis machines that can measure 12 components in a blood sample at the rate of 60 samples per hour. There are more differences than similarities between the pharmaceutical industry and the industries involved in the production of devices, medical supplies and equipment. Here are some of the major differences.

Perhaps the most significant difference is the way in which the consumer pays for the products involved. Consumers paid directly 85 percent of the more than $6 billion spent at retail for 1.5 billion drug prescriptions filled in 1971. In contrast some mode of indirect payment was involved for 84 percent of the consumable supplies and equipment used during illnesses in the same year. Prosthetic devices, including eyeglasses, which are paid for directly, accounted for the remaining 16 percent. Supplies are said to be paid for indirectly when they are part of a consolidated bill presented by a hospital or clinic or when they are part of a bill paid by an insurance carrier or other third party. In either case the patient is usually unaware of the details.

A corollary of the mode of payment leads to the second major difference between the drug houses and the makers of medical supplies: the degree of product visibility. The general public is aware of and concerned about such issues as the safety of oral contraceptives, price-fixing in antibiotics and the debate over brand-name v. generic-name prescription writing. The public has little or no interest, however, in such matters as proof of safety and effectiveness of equipment used for patient care or the unnecessary duplication of costly equipment by hospitals located in the same area. One thinks, for example, of the fad for installing hyperbaric chambers in hospital operating rooms in the mid-1960's. Costing upward of $100,000 per installation, their value to the patient undergoing surgery now appears marginal.

Product visibility, or lack of it, helps to explain the third major difference between the part of the industry that produces drugs and the part that produces supplies and equipment. Whereas the Government subjects drug makers to heavy regulation, it has only recently begun to regulate the makers of medical supplies and equipment.

The fourth major difference between the two parts of the industry is in profitability. The pharmaceutical houses out-perform all other major American industries in net profit after taxes as a percent of stockholders' equity. The drug companies regularly show a return of about 18 percent, a figure two-thirds higher than the average rate of return for all manufacturing concerns in the decade 1960–1970. Although the consolidated data are not available for direct comparison, it is evident from the annual reports of the major companies in the medical supplies and equipment business that their rates of return are closer to the industrial average of 11 percent than to the drug companies' 18 percent. These, then, are the two major segments of the medical business: one highly visible, highly profitable and highly controversial, the other almost hidden from view, returning only average profits and making few "waves." Let us now take a closer look at the two segments.

The pharmaceutical industry manufactures two major classes of products: proprietary drugs sold freely over the counter and ethical drugs, which require a prescription. Ethical pharmaceuticals are further subdivided into brand-name and generic products. The former are patented products manufactured by the larger companies; the latter are substances on which the patent has usually expired and that bear a uniform chemical name regardless of the source.

In 1971, according to surveys conducted by the magazine *Drug Topics,* the dollar volume of all packaged medicines sold at retail without a prescription was $2.9 billion. Of this total cough and cold "remedies" accounted for $619 million, headache nostrums for $600 million and mouthwashes and gargles for $240 million [*see illustration on next page*]. Many observers question the desirability of this traffic in drugs that are mostly marginal in their effectiveness. Although

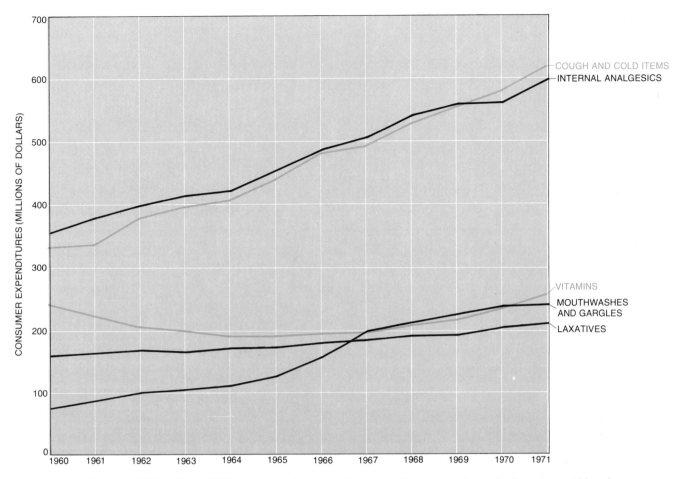

U.S. SALES OF NONPRESCRIPTION DRUGS increased 67 percent between 1960 and 1971. Total retail sales of all packaged medicines in 1971 was $2.9 billion. Year in, year out cough and cold "remedies" and internal analgesics (aspirin and the like) account for about 40 percent of the total sales volume. Although consumption of vitamins approximately doubled in the period, dollar volume remained almost constant because vitamins became cheaper. Figures are from surveys published by the magazine *Drug Topics*.

they are heavily advertised as being capable of relieving and even curing various target ailments, the claims are rarely supported by objective studies. The Federal Trade Commission has begun to look closely at the curative claims made for these over-the-counter drugs in television and newspaper advertisements.

Meanwhile the prescription drug industry is enjoying an unbroken rise in sales. The value of ethical-drug shipments in 1971 was $4.11 billion, an increase of more than 100 percent in 10 years, with no leveling off in sight [*see the illustration on page 122*]. If Congress were to enact some kind of comprehensive national health-insurance plan that would include payment for prescription drugs, total sales could jump 20 to 25 percent almost overnight.

I shall leave it to other authors in this issue to question whether Americans really need 1.5 billion drug prescriptions per year or an average of 20 per family. I shall limit my remarks to the way the industry uses its sales dollars.

It is estimated that the ethical-drug houses currently spend $1.2 billion per year on advertising and promotion. This represents about $1 in every $4 they receive for their products at wholesale and is nearly four times what they spend annually on research and development. Virtually none of the marketing expenditures are directed at the consumer who buys the product. They are directed at the physician who writes the prescription and at the pharmacist who, with increasing frequency, is in a position to select the brand when the prescription is written generically or when it allows him to substitute one brand for another.

Since the marketing costs come to about $4,000 per physician per year they are deemed excessive by many critics of the industry. The $1.2-billion figure includes the salaries of more than 21,000 "detail men," each of whom costs the industry an estimated $35,000 per year; their sole job is to make periodic calls on physicians, pharmacists and hospital purchasing agents to push their firm's products. Also included in the $1.2 billion are such costs as advertising in medical journals, exhibits at medical conventions, direct-mail pieces (including physicians' samples), seminars, educational films,

brochures and the practice of allowing wholesalers, retailers and hospitals to return unsold merchandise for credit. How essential these expenditures are is a matter of judgment. That they add significantly to the nation's drug bill is undisputable.

During the past five years research costs in the pharmaceutical industry have averaged close to 6 percent of net sales, a figure comparable to that in other high-technology industries. In the same period the return on research investments, as measured by new products, has shown a steady decline. The decline followed the passage of the Kefauver-Harris amendments to the Federal Food, Drug, and Cosmetic Act of 1962, which substantially increased the Food and Drug Administration's regulating authority with respect to the testing and marketing of new drugs. The peak for new chemical entities (63) was reached in 1959; the peaks for new combinations (253) and new dosage forms (109) had been reached a year earlier [*see top illustration on page 125*]. By requiring that new drugs be efficacious as well as safe, the Kefauver-Harris amend-

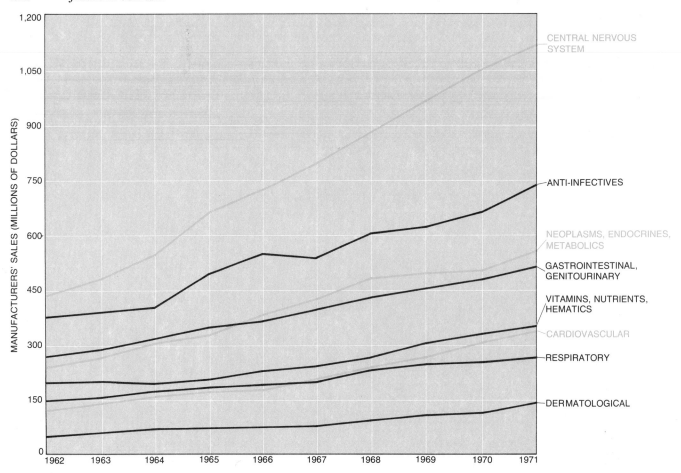

SALES OF PRESCRIPTION, OR ETHICAL, DRUGS more than doubled between 1962 and 1971, increasing from $1.89 billion to $4.11 billion in wholesale value. The sharpest increases were exhibited by cardiovascular drugs (up 173 percent) and by drugs that affect the central nervous system, the category that includes tranquilizers and other mood-modifying drugs (up 136 percent). Oral contraceptives are included in the classification "Neoplasms, endocrines, metabolics," which increased about 130 percent.

ments accelerated the decline in all three categories of new products. With 5,558 new products entering the marketplace between 1950 and 1962 the country needed not more combinations, new dosage forms and duplicate products but more effective drugs.

In spite of some predictions the amendments have not stifled drug research. The quest for new drugs continues apace. The total industry outlay for research and development exceeds $500 million per year, and the Federal Government spends $1.75 billion on drug testing alone.

Production costs in the pharmaceutical industry average a third of the manufacturer's sales dollar. The most significant portion of this expenditure, however, is related not to the cost of raw materials or to the manufacturing process itself but rather to the highly complex quality-control procedures required by Federal law. More than 8,000 workers, 16 percent of the industry's work force, are engaged in quality control.

Profitability has long been the hallmark of the pharmaceutical industry. Year after year the industry ranks first or second in after-tax income as a percentage of net worth. This profitability has been maintained by the drug industry even though drug prices have not climbed as rapidly as consumer prices in general. The drug industry has been able to limit price increases thanks in large part to the high degree of automatic control achieved in its manufacturing processes. At the same time the absence of price competition for most products has ensured continued high profits.

When the pharmaceutical industry is called on to defend its large profit margins, it responds that it is in a high-risk business in which vast sums are spent on research with little or no guarantee of return. Spokesmen for the drug industry often compare the search for new drugs with the drilling of wildcat wells in the oil industry. The fact is that during the past 25 years no major pharmaceutical house has been forced out of business. As one economist said in testimony before the Senate Select Committee on Small Business: "The high profitability reflects the absence of competition; the stability of profits demonstrates the absence of risk to investors. If risks were to exist, one would expect to see the high gains of some firms accompanied by occasional losses—to themselves or to others—but such evidence of risk is virtually nonexistent."

The industry's profitability has been maintained also in the face of rising Government interest in and control of its activities. Federal interest was aroused in the era of Theodore Roosevelt, when the blatant claims of many makers of patent medicines led to calls for Government regulation. Apart from the fact that the claims were often misleading and even dangerous, many of the nostrums contained opium derivatives, with the result that many people unwittingly became addicted to the drug. Harvey W. Wiley, a chemist in the Department of Agriculture, was one of the leaders in the effort to bring patent medicines under control. It was not until the publication of Upton Sinclair's novel *The Jungle*, however, that Congress responded by passing the Food and Drug Act of 1906. From this modest beginning the Federal role in drug regulation has grown to its present level. In each instance drug legislation granting new authority was precipitated by some crisis affecting the consumer.

In 1938, for example, it was the elixir of sulfanilamide disaster, in which the use of ethylene glycol as a solvent by a chemist with the S. E. Massengill Company led to the death of more than 100 persons, most of them small children. Congress swiftly enacted a law requiring that drugs be proved safe prior to marketing. Such legislation had been sought by the Executive Branch of the Government each year since 1933, only to be beaten back each time in Congress through the efforts of the drug-industry lobby.

In 1961, when the thalidomide tragedy struck in Europe, Richardson-Merrell, a major U.S. pharmaceutical manufacturer, had a new-drug application for thalidomide pending before the Food and Drug Administration. Thanks to the vigilance of Frances Oldham Kelsey, a physician and pharmacologist on the FDA staff, the application was held up and ultimately never issued. Congress again acted swiftly by passing the Ke-fauver-Harris amendments, which provided the FDA with an entire range of new authorities, including the requirement that all new drugs must be proved not only safe but also effective before being allowed to enter the marketplace. The FDA was also empowered to require periodic reports from manufacturers; to require that ethical-drug advertising be honest, with sufficient balance to give the physician information about a drug's side effects and contraindications as well as its potential benefits; to require immediate reporting of any un-

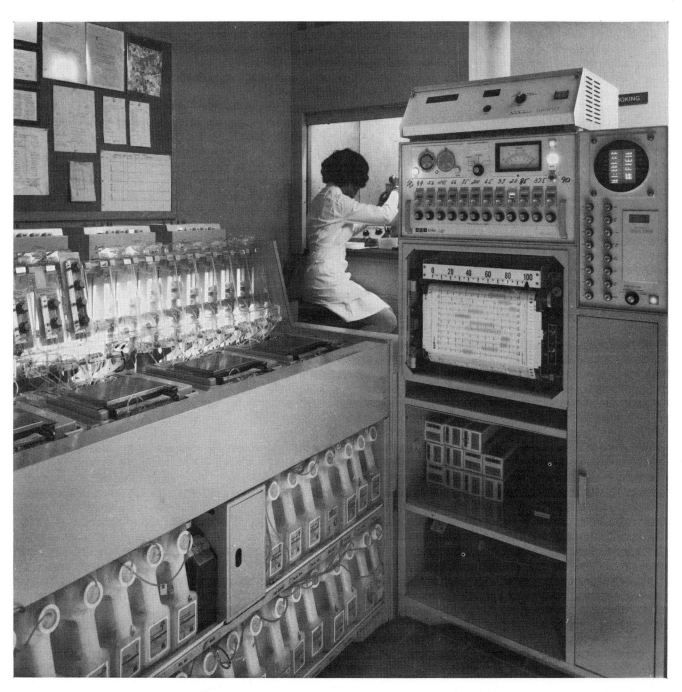

AUTOMATIC ANALYSIS OF BLOOD SAMPLES is carried out by a $100,000 machine built by the Technicon Corporation. The instrument can analyze blood specimens for 12 different components at the rate of 60 specimens per hour. Components commonly determined include calcium, inorganic phosphate, urea nitrogen, glucose, uric acid, albumin, total protein, cholesterol, alkaline phosphatase and lactic dehydrogenase. The instrument shown here is in the New York City laboratory of the Life Extension Institute.

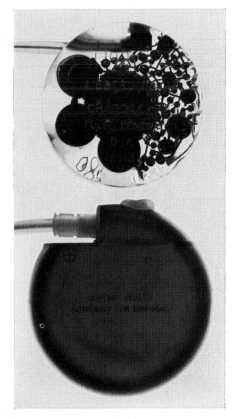

IMPLANTABLE PACEMAKERS for the heart are among the many medical devices not yet brought under the control of the Food and Drug Administration. It is estimated that 50,000 Americans will receive pacemaker implants this year. The two devices shown here are made by Medtronic, Inc., of Minneapolis. The unit at top, which uses a chemical power source, has an expected life of two to three years. Unit at bottom, which runs on plutonium 238, may last 10 years. Each weighs about five ounces.

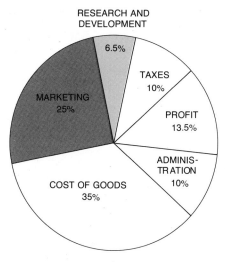

RESEARCH AND DEVELOPMENT
6.5%
TAXES 10%
MARKETING 25%
PROFIT 13.5%
ADMINIS-TRATION 10%
COST OF GOODS 35%

BREAKDOWN OF SALES DOLLAR is estimated for 1968 for 17 leading pharmaceutical houses. Although the industry takes pride in its large investment in research and development (some $400 million in 1968), the amount spent on marketing and promotion is nearly four times larger. The industry is second only to mining in profitability.

usual side effects during development work, and to review all drugs marketed between 1938 and 1962 to determine their efficacy as well as their safety.

Some observers believe that the pharmaceutical industry is now overregulated and that bureaucratic interference with the industry has reached such a level that the American public is being denied certain drugs available overseas. The University of Chicago economist Milton Friedman has recently made this point forcefully, and with much publicity, by charging that FDA regulations are keeping important new drugs off the American market and that the U.S. is falling behind the rest of the world in the development of new drugs. Calling for repeal of the Kefauver-Harris amendments, Friedman pointed to the availability in Europe of two new drugs for heart patients, Practolol and Oxprenolol, as prime examples of why the present system should be changed.

Friedman's allegations were effectively refuted during recent Senate hearings by spokesmen from three organizations that rarely find themselves in total agreement about anything: the Food and Drug Administration, the American Medical Association and the Pharmaceutical Manufacturers Association. Spokesmen for these groups, along with a number of prominent heart and cancer specialists, made it quite clear that even though the U.S. has the most demanding requirements of any nation in the world, all safe and effective drugs, or their equivalents, are available here. (Practolol and Oxprenolol are not deemed safe.)

The companies that manufacture medical supplies, devices and equipment might be termed the hidden, or at least the unknown, segment of the medical business. When the patient is billed for blood tests or X rays, it probably does not occur to him that part of the fee is used to offset the purchase price of expensive analytical instruments or an X-ray camera. And who even cares that the doctor's bill must cover the cost of tongue depressors, Band-Aids, thermometers, disposable hypodermic syringes and the almost countless other impedimenta of medical practice?

In spite of their low profile, the companies that make these medical goods are enjoying the sharply rising expenditures on health care. For example, manufacturers of surgical dressings and instruments have annual sales of more than $500 million. This amount includes $163 million for adhesive tape, $127 million for compresses, gauze and other dress-

ings, $88 million for elastic bandages and rolls containing plaster of Paris for making casts and $30 million for cotton balls. Sales of surgical instruments come to about $120 million per year.

Manufacturers of other kinds of medical supplies have annual sales of more than $2 billion. Sales are expected to reach $2.9 billion by 1975 and $4.2 billion by 1980. Products under this heading include anesthetics, parenteral solutions, syringes and needles, sutures, laboratory ware and reagents, thermometers, stethoscopes, sphygmomanometers, medical linen and X-ray supplies. (More square feet of photographic film are consumed in making X rays than are used by the motion-picture industry, which has recently led the Eastman Kodak Company to introduce a system for copying the standard 14-by-17-inch X-ray image on a "chip" about two inches square so that the silver in the original large negative can be recycled.)

The introduction of new technology, much of it made possible by solid-state electronics, has led to a sharp rise in the sales of medical and hospital equipment. The magazine *Electronics* predicts, for example, that sales will increase more than 50 percent between 1970 and 1975: from $530 million to $832 million. Sales of patient-monitoring systems will nearly triple in the same period: from $29 million to $80 million.

Sizable increases are also predicted for sales of such laboratory equipment as automatic clinical chemistry systems, blood-bank equipment, blood analyzers, chromatography systems, electrolyte-measuring instruments, automatic blood-cell counters, electron and light microscopes and spectrophotometers. Sales of these items, which were less than $200 million in 1968, may reach $380 million in 1975 and exceed $570 million in 1980, according to *Electronics*.

The use of new plastics and alloys has led to great advances in such surgical implants as artificial joints, bone plates, pins and arterial grafts. It is estimated that 100,000 arterial grafts will be inserted this year, along with 45,000 heart valves and 200,000 cerebrospinal-fluid shunts (mechanical devices for relieving excess aqueous pressure within the brain). It is estimated that 100,000 Americans are now equipped with electronic heart pacemakers and that 50,000 new installations will be made this year. More than three million women have now been fitted with intrauterine contraceptive devices (IUD's) in the form of rings, coils, loops, bows, springs and spirals.

During the remainder of the decade

one can expect major progress in the development of assistive, prosthetic and corrective devices, such as "radar" aids for the blind and artificial larynxes. Sales of devices in this category are expected to reach $640 million by 1975 and $890 million by 1980.

Many observers believe the medical-supply industry is in the same position as the drug industry was in before the enactment of the 1938 legislation. There has been an enormous proliferation of medical devices (a recent FDA survey counted 12,000 devices made by 1,100 companies), but no Federal agency has yet been given the responsibility for determining either their safety or their efficacy. The International Organization for Standardization has been pressing its member countries to exercise greater control over devices with the greatest potential for doing harm, particularly surgical implants. At the same time the FDA has been asking Congress to increase its control over the manufacture and sale of medical devices of all kinds.

In recent testimony before a Congressional subcommittee the then Acting FDA Commissioner Sherwin Gardner noted that under the limited powers granted the agency in 1938 most of its effort, until recently at least, had been devoted to removing obviously dangerous products from the market and controlling the promotion of "quack type" devices. "Because existing law imposes no statutory requirements for FDA to review the safety and effectiveness of medical devices prior to marketing," Gardner testified, "FDA has the burden of proof and must accumulate evidence sufficient to assure that it can sustain a court action."

An indication of the seriousness of the problem is that, even with such limited powers, the FDA in the first three months of this year seized more than 300 devices, ordered the recall of 35 different kinds of device (including several hundred heart pacemakers) and issued more than 1,800 advisory opinions (letters of warning or caution to manufacturers). A bill that is currently before Congress would enable the agency to require all manufacturers of medical devices to be registered with the FDA, to disclose all complaints received, to maintain records and submit reports (including clinical studies of safety and efficacy) and to recall, replace or repair defective devices. One would hope that adequate control legislation will for once in this country be enacted on its merits and not in response to a tragedy.

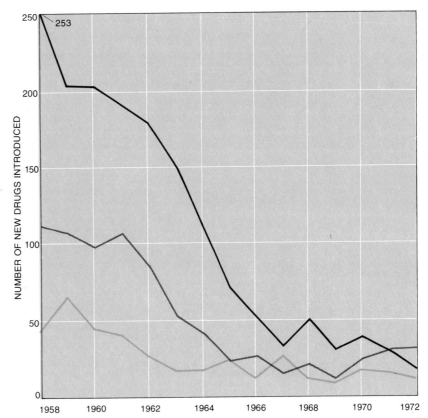

INTRODUCTION OF NEW DRUGS reached a peak a few years before Congress passed the Kefauver-Harris amendments that made the FDA responsible for seeing that new drugs are efficacious as well as safe. New chemical entities (*colored curve*) reached a peak in 1959. New combinations (*black curve*) and new dosage forms (*gray*) peaked a year earlier.

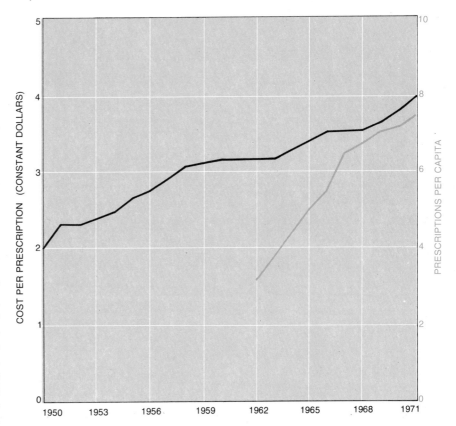

NUMBER OF PRESCRIPTIONS PER CAPITA (*colored curve*) has increased 150 percent in the past 10 years. Prescriptions dispensed in hospitals (3.4 per capita in 1971) are not included. Between 1950 and 1971 the average cost of a prescription (*black curve*) almost exactly doubled. In the same period the U.S. consumer price index rose only 68 percent.